Prof. Dr. Elmar Wienecke

Performance Explosion in Sports
An Anti-Doping Concept

Revolutionary New Findings
in the Area of Micronutrient Therapy

Training Continuity
Training Optimization
Injury Prevention through
Personalized Micronutrients

Meyer & Meyer Sport

Original title: Leistungsexplosion im Sport
© 2011 by Meyer & Meyer Verlag

Translated by Petra Haynes
AAA Translation, St. Louis, Missouri, USA
www.AAATranslation.com

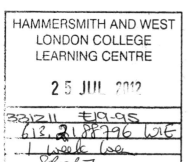
Performance Explosion in Sports –
An Anti-Doping Concept
Prof. Dr. Elmar Wienecke
Maidenhead: Meyer & Meyer Sport (UK) Ltd., 2011
ISBN: 978-1-84126-330-4

© 2011 by Meyer & Meyer Verlag, Aachen
Auckland, Beirut, Budapest, Cairo, Cape Town, Dubai, Indianapolis,
Kindberg, Maidenhead, Sydney, Olten, Singapore, Tehran, Toronto
Member of the World
Sport Publishers' Association (WSPA)
www.w-s-p-a.org
Printing by: B.O.S.S Druck und Medien GmbH
ISBN 978-1-84126-330-4
E-Mail: info@m-m-sports.com
www.m-m-sports.com

Contents

Various documents and material in this book can be downloaded
as PDF templates and worksheets from the publisher's website at
www.m-m- sports.com/extras/performance_explosion.
The download code can be found at the respective places in the book.

Photo: Comstock

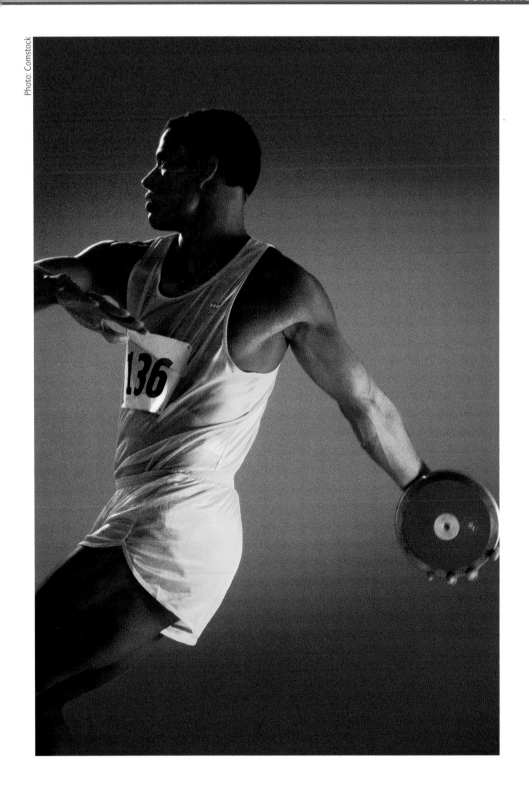

Preface

We are all familiar with this: a twinge, a pang, or any number of other little discomforts that frequently prevent the athlete from achieving his optimal potential. But even serious injuries without external force, such as torn ligaments in the knee, shoulder or ankle, have dramatically increased in recent years in all sports.

The dream of winning the championship, the need for success as an acknowledgment of personal strength, the lucrative financial offers, all have resulted in athletes increasingly using banned substances to create a competitive edge for themselves, both in recreational as well as performance sports. The doping problem extends to all sports. A former competitive athlete claims that nowadays winning is impossible without these substances. What an absurd misjudgment!

In fact, the key to effective injury prophylaxis and possible performance explosion lies with simple optimized preventative measures. The engine of a car won't run without gas, and it's the same with the performance development and injury prophylaxis of athletes. Athletes are unable to meet their full potential without micronutrients. There exists a connection between the cellular nutrient con-centration and degeneration of bradytrophe tissue (ligaments, snears, cartilage). This will be confirmed with special parameters (i.a. pyridinium crosslinks). However, to date scientists deny these correlations. According to statements by international scientists, "little knowledge" exists on the positive effects of a specific micronutrient supply in athletes. It is still in its infancy.

In the past ten years, our institute SALUTO and its cooperation partners have examined 9,150 athletes (i.a. European champions, world champions) and 6.434 recreational athletes from all different sports, and by means of a unique European prevention program for young star-athletes (national level youth and junior team handball players), were able to acquire new and highly interesting findings in the area of micronutrient therapy. Of note were the dramatic cellular micronutrient deficiencies of top athletes and many recreational athletes. Ambitious athletes live dangerously in the truest sense of the word, without the "optimal" fuel (micronutrient supply).

Contrary to previous findings from interdisciplinary research in sports medicine, sports and nutritional science, our present research results show that a good diet and an optimal customized micronutrient concentration clearly reduce the risk of injury, increase the athletes' performance, and can lead to performance consistency.

Together let us delve into the fascinating world of micronutrient therapy in athletes. The goal is a definite performance increase by tapping into existing potential through natural means. Do not rely on the dietary methods of yesterday and specifically implement your own anti-doping concept. A condensed version of many of the findings, background information and practical tips introduced here can be found in the appendix or can be downloaded as a PDF file (available from the publisher with corresponding code number).

Clean, injury-free and successful sports are no myth or fairytale but can become a reality!

Regards,
Prof. Dr. Elmar Wienecke
Sports Scientist

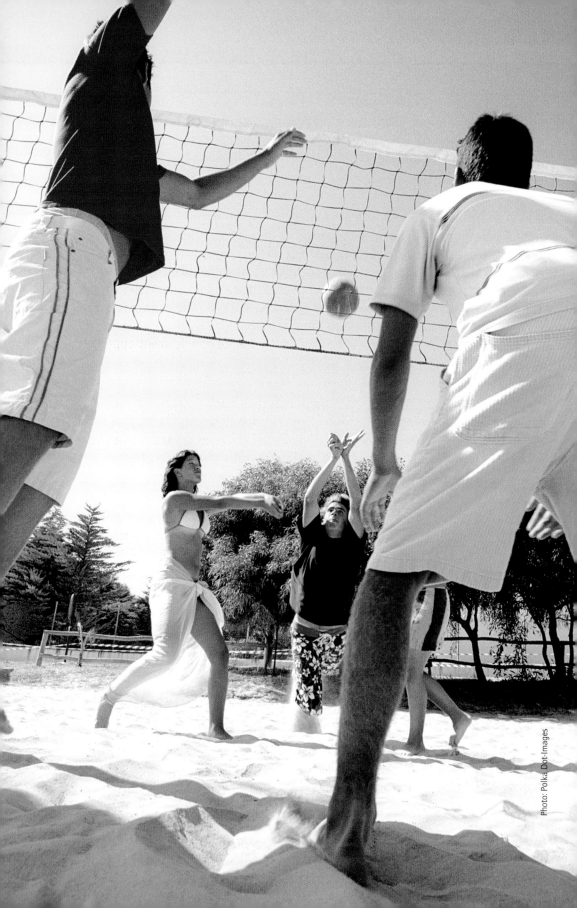

1 Introduction

1.1 The Anti-Doping Concept – the personalized micronutrient formulation

Athletes live dangerously! The higher the training intensity and volume of competitive athletes, the higher the danger of training interruption due to frequent infections and injuries to the connective tissue (ligaments, tendons and cartilage). Of the 9,150 competitive and 6.434 recreational athletes examined by SALUTO, 72% of all injuries were sustained without external force. These are injuries to various connective tissue structures of the tendon-ligament apparatus and the musculature.

There are obvious correlations between the concentration of cellular micronutrients (amino acids, vitamins, minerals, trace elements), the degeneration of bradytrophic tissue structures (ligaments, tendons, various cartilage substances), injury susceptibility (see pg. 101, 102, 108), the status of the immune system, and the performance consistency of competitive athletes.

Definite links can be seen between optimal micronutrient formulation and the repression of inflammatory and degenerative changes in competitive athletes with the aid of special laboratory parameters such as COMP (cartilege oligometric matrix protein) and the pyridinium crosslinks. The athletes taking the customized micronutrient formulation clearly exhibit lower COMP values after four months than the group of competitive athletes that took doses of micronutrients according to DGE guidelines. The results of the pyridinium crosslinks in urine show a similar effect (see pg. 108).

In our experience structural changes in the tendon and ligament apparatus and the various cartilage structures can only be seen several years later with the aid of MRT images (and not, as was previously thought, after 4 to 8 months). Future long term testing of athletes with the aid of MRT images and the listed special blood parameters will have to confirm these correlations.

1.2   What's so special about the anti-doping concept

The application of the newest diagnostic methods to diagnose deficiencies or rather the micronutrient requirements, even on the cellular level, as well as micronutrient supplementation tailored to the individual athlete (only made possible thereby) or his current situation make the anti-doping concept special. There are many fairytales and myths regarding the necessity of customized micronutrient supplementation for competitive athletes. Details can be found on pages 16-20.

The results of a scientific analysis of athletes at the Olympics in Athens in 2004, showed that based on available results no general substitution requirements existed in competitive athletes. According to the authors, the ascertained deficiencies are not a sport-specific problem. Based on today's knowledge (completed projects and clinical studies, see pg. 44-50), this assertion is incomprehensible. The tests in question were performed only in the serum and not at the cellular level. In addition these nutritional analyses do not take into account the verifiable reductions of micronutrient concentrations due to the greenhouse effect (see pg. 40-42).

There is a direct link between the high injury risk in competitive athletes and an optimal micronutrient supply. Without "optimal fuel" ambitious athletes live dangerously in the truest sense of the word. The long-term negative consequences of intensive athletic exertion, and the resulting increased vulnerability of the various listed connective tissue structuresparticularly demonstrate the urgent need for a customized micronutrient formulation. The dosage recommendations clearly differ from the previously postulated guidelines by the DGE (German Nutrition Society) and the DGSP (German Society for Sports Medicine and Prevention) (see pg. 246-269, Tables 29-32). Numerous competitive tennis players, many professional athletes from different sports, but also team athletes such as the youth and junior players of the German national handball team have been benefitting from these specific customized micronutrient formulations for the past four years (see pg. 204-207) with proven positive results. Intracellular and additional blood and nutrition analyses are necessary for the composition of the formulations. The creation of the individual micronutrient formulation is based primarily on preventative considerations and relies on a worldwide unique database.

1.3   Fairytales and myths
about micronutrient therapy for athletes

1.   Scientists (i.a. clinical nutritionists and sports doctors) claim:
      Supplementary micronutrients for athletes are unnecessary; that
      assertion is simply daylight robbery by the micronutrient industry.
      Optimal nutrition is sufficient!

This statement does not apply. After personally conducting clinical studies and
projects (see pg. 44-50) it became apparent that the micronutrient requirements
of athletes with only a three-hour weekly endurance training session are not met
in spite of a balanced diet. However, the appropriate testers are essential here.
Routine blood serum tests do not provide information about the particular
micronutrient concentration (see pg. 34-40).

Scientific research during recent years and personal inquiries to American
biologists (see pg. 42) show that the greenhouse effect in particular has caused a
tremendous increase in CO_2, resulting in a fundamental loss of nutrients in our
plants. We must correct the present perception of many nutritional scientists who
have been extremely critical of the customized use of micronutrients by athletes.

It is, however, also true that the micronutrient industry has a large commercial
interest in bringing their products to market through clever marketing strategies. It
is particularly important to pay attention to the quality and dosage of products.
Most critical are the personal requirements of the individual athlete rather than
the overall supply of the recommended dosages propagated by the micronutrient
industry. In addition the required micronutrients must be consistent with the Anti-
Doping Commission guidelines.

2.   A scientific analysis conducted with athletes at the Athens Olympics in
      2004, (see Faude, O. et al, 2005), came to the conclusion that there is no
      general substitution requirement for top athletes. According to the
      authors any detected deficiencies are not sport-specific problems.

Based on today's knowledge (completed clinical study, see pg. 47-49), this
statement is not comprehensible. The former tests were done on serum only and
not at the cellular level. In addition these nutritional analyses do not take into
account the proven reductions of micronutrient concentrations due to the
greenhouse effect.

Fairytales and myths in micronutrient therapy

Statement: in Leistungssport, May 19, 2005
(Faude, Fuhrmann, Herrmann, Kindermann & Urhausen)

Results from the scientific analysis
of 23 athletes after the Athens Olympics

- General substitution requirements do not exist.

- Diagnosed under-supply of some micronutrients
  is not a sport-specific problem.

- Detection of individual micronutrient deficiencies:
  nutrition analyses are better than blood analyses.

Fig. 1

3. Micronutrients can be a substitute for an unbalanced (poor) diet!

This statement is definitely false! A balanced diet according to the guidelines of the international Nutrition Society is the basis for the absorption of individual micronutrient formulations into the gastrointestinal tract. If the athlete thinks he can relieve his guilty conscience by consuming specific micronutrients, only a small percentage of these will actually end up in his bloodstream.

4. No topic is more hotly debated in the scientific community than the specific use of micronutrients in sports. Current micronutrient recommendations for athletes are still in their infancy. There is limited knowledge about side effects of multiple micronutrient concentrations!

The following assertion by international scientists is correct: If medical science wants to develop more reasonable and effective prophylaxis and therapy strategies in the future, it will not be able to avoid the mitochondria. In a consensus paper on genomic stability through micronutrients (Fenech et al, 2001) international scientists summarized their findings:

- Current micronutrient recommendations are based on the prevention of deficiency diseases.

- There is limited knowledge about multiple simultaneous micronutrient deficiencies.

- Unknown interactions with gene and thus enzyme polymorphisms (e.g., α-Tocopherol inhibits gluthatione-S-transferase)

- There is no substantiated knowledge about the mitochondrial genome, its oxidative stress and the significance of micronutrients.

Even at that time, international scientists were of the opinion that higher doses of individually composed micronutrient formulations could support the maintenance of connective tissue structures (tendon-ligament apparatus, stability of various cartilage structures) in competitive athletes or even in cases of chronic illness.

5. Higher doses of micronutrient formulations are unnecessary and should be rejected!

This assertion is false! True is: To date there is a lack of sports medicine and exercise physiology data for the practical review of the clinical relevance of present dosage recommendations. The presently recommended use is only derived from basic considerations about the relationship between energy use and increased nutrient requirements (per: Dickhut, pg. 496, 2007). However, this does not mean that the specific use of individually higher dosage recommendations for athletes should be rejected. Based on our findings, the micronutrient requirements for energy supply, particularly during intensive training and competition phases, is clearly higher than previously thought. The verifiable reductions of micronutrient concentrations in plants due to the greenhouse effect and the considerably lowered injury risk in competitive athletes due to targeted individual micronutrient formulations, are indications of an increasing demand.

6. Micronutrients have no verifiable impact on the risk of injury and infection in athletes!

This assertion is false! Our experience in the care of recreational and competitive athletes shows the necessity and efficiency of the targeted use of higher-dose micronutrient formulations for the athletes' immune system and a definite lowering of the injury risk. Those athletes who received specific micronutrient formulations were able to verifiably perform their training program largely without injury or infection. The training continuity of the athletes who received individually prepared micronutrient formulations was clearly noticeable compared to the group of athletes who did not receive micronutrient formulations. This was done over a period of two years (see pg. 100-102). The accompanying analysis of the athletes' diet in both groups conformed to the guidelines of the German Nutrition Society, but also to those of international standards.

The newly developed laboratory parameter COMP (cartilege oligometric matrix protein) and the pyridinium crosslinks in urine show initial correlations between optimal micronutrient formulation and infectious (degenerative) changes in performance athletes. Personal initial examination findings in competitive athletes with the aid of very expensive MRT imaging show possible correlations between long-term micronutrient deficiencies and the strain on many connective tissue structures (degenerative changes of tendon-ligament apparatus and cartilage structure) only after approximately three years upon completion of a planned innovative pilot project with competitive athletes.

7. **A lot helps a lot! The higher the dose of a micronutrient concentration the more effective it is.**

This assertion is false. Higher doses of vitamins, trace elements and minerals can have adverse effects. Consumption of high amounts of niacin can verifiably cause allergic skin reactions. Selenium taken in higher concentration, for instance more than 200 µg for an extended period of time, can lead to toxic reactions. A customized micronutrient formulation can be prepared depending on the diet, the cellular micronutrient concentration, the training intensity and the training volume of the individual athlete. Too much magnesium can, for instance, reduce the ability to absorb calcium.

8. **A blanket approach to supplying micronutrients for competitive athletes must be rejected. Currently used dosage recommendations are frequently insufficient for athletes.**

All qualitative suppliers of micronutrient concentration products – whether they sell natural juices or various combination preparations- point to the high availability of their organic products. The more natural, the more effective is the tenor of their advertising slogan. But due to dosage guidelines all of these products can only cover the athlete's basic requirements.

It must be noted that these criteria have to comply with the Ant-Doping Commission and cannot be contaminated with other substances. This risk can be avoided with, for instance, a product quality standard from pharmacies that can incorporate their micronutrients as a "building block" into a matrix through a patented process, such as is ideally done with HCK® formulations. Additionally, in our experience the specific use of high-quality proteins with their many amino acids is absolutely necessary for the stabilization of connective tissue structures. The micronutrient recommendations that are to date being propagated by many sports and nutrition scientists will be reformed by innovative, long-term accompanying analyses. A special cellular analysis of micronutrients for the creation of these formulations (particularly for a frequently diagnosed latent hypofuntion of the thyroid (see pg. 146-149) has been suggested. A supply of micronutrients can of course also be achieved with various combinations of single-agent preparations in specially adapted formulations and a temporally varied intake mode.

9. Accurate diagnostics are the nuts and bolts of micronutrient therapy in athletes

The creation of micronutrient formulations also presupposes optimal diagnostics. There are very few institutions with the ability to conduct these expensive cellular analyses, and even fewer experts who are able toadequately interpret the measured results for athletes. Our institute SALUTO has access to a databank that is currently based on 9,150 athletes from all sports. Thus element determination in serum does not allow for reliable conclusions with respect to mineral, vitamin and trace element balance. Important biochemical mechanisms of action of elements take place primarily on the cellular level. Determination of the element concentration from serum can therefore offer no information about cellular processes (see pg. 34-40).

The exchange between extra and intracellular space is regulated by complex autologous mechanisms. The concentration of essential elements in serum is kept as constant as possible. Autologous reserves are mobilized to maintain the serum level, should the micronutrient supply (vitamins, minerals, etc.) be insufficient to do so. This is why serum deficiencies are often recognized too late or not at all.

10. Sufficient amounts of vitamins, minerals, trace elements do not create world champions.

The first assumption is absolutely correct. A sufficient basic supply makes it possible to optimally utilize an athlete's performance potential. However, our experience in recent years shows that an optimal basic supply of basic micronutrients has lead to optimal training continuity (marked by a distinctly low infection risk) and improved maintenance of many connective tissue functions (tendon-ligament apparatus) (see pg. 101, 102). After three years of individual micronutrient formulation use in youth and junior national team handball players from the German Team Handball Federation within the scope of the unique European prevention concept, and the development of the players' holistic development potential (from the state of their teeth to character-building techniques promoting increased personal responsibility), the players report a distinctly lower injury rate, improved ability for regeneration after intensive physical strain and thus a long-term increase in performance. All of these different puzzle pieces lead to the Division A-youth team's European championship victory in 2008, and the junior team's world championship victory in 2009. But the specific, long-term use of customized micronutrient formulations has also verifiably improved the injury risk and thereby the performance of many other competitive athletes. Performance athletes live dangerously in the truest sense of the word.

1.4 Injury risk and performance fluctuation due to cellular deficiencies of micronutrients – examples from different sports

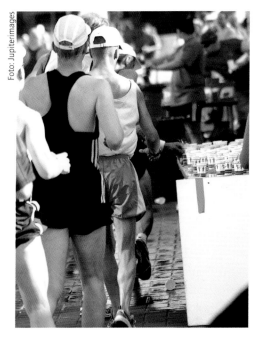

Foto: Jupiterimages

Today no one doubts that competitive athletes bear high health risks. Thus the sports magazine Sportbild stridently concluded in November 2009: "Germany's 184,800.000 Euro soccer stars breaking down! Never has it been this bad! And this in spite of many personal trainers and optimal medical care!" Like the top athlete Paula Radcliffe, who suffered a fatigue fracture in the left femoral prior to the Peking Olympics, it is not uncommon for competitive athletes from all disciplines (soccer, team handball, etc) to be affected by these types of injuries without external force.

Provocative assumptions

- Micronutrient deficiencies can cause a variety of long-term malaise (fatigue, performance fluctuation and injuries).

- Iodine and selenium deficiencies can cause drastic thyroid problems in performance athletes, resulting in extreme performance fluctuations and injuries.

- Micronutrient deficiencies lead to decreased regeneration ability and lack of concentration.

- Athletes are at high risk for infection due to micronutrient deficiencies and therefore a lack of training continuity.

Our results from 1994-2009, with a total of 15.584 recreational and competitive athletes showed a high injury risk without external force of more than 68%. More than half the athletes sustain hitherto inexplicable injuries (muscle injuries or even tears, many fatigue fractures, severe infection propensity in competitive athletes, etc.)

Early warning system for endurance athletes reveals sensational results

i.a., a new study by MRT radiologists (German Radiology Society) of triathletes done with the aid of magnetic resonance tomography before and after the 2007 triathlon in Kärnten, Austria, showed:

- **A dramatic trend in micro-injuries of the knee and ankle joints, muscle edema, inflammation of the Achilles tendon, etc., in recreational, competitive and top athletes;**

- **Micro-injuries worsened all the way to fractures (fatigue fractures, etc.) after competitive exertion.**

Fig. 2

How we tested

Of a total 1,150 athletes (N = 559) received an individual micronutrient formulation; the other group of athletes (N = 591) received no micronutrients. Each of these athletes underwent biomechanical functional analyses of all muscle groups, special cellular blood analyses (portions of the immune system), neuromuscular coordination tests of knees and ankles, video and structural analyses.

Each athlete received personal training plans based on the biomechanical functional analyses we conducted, to optimize their individual performance, particularly if cases of muscular imbalance.

Initial misalignments or stresses and strains could be remedied with the aid of video and detailed structural analyses. Additional risk factors were previously minimized via special dental examinations (particularly microbiological diagnostics) and preventative measures.

An overview of the results

The high injury rate to the tendon-ligament apparatus and the muscular system, but also training absences due to infections, showed the link to the striking cellular micronutrient deficiencies (minerals, trace elements, vitamins, amino acids) in 591 competitive athletes, measured over a three-year period.

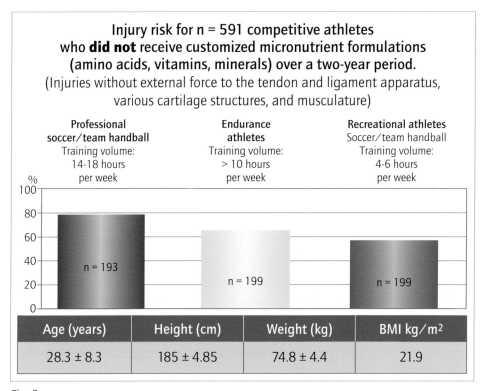

Fig. 3

Due to the specific supply of individual micronutrient formulations and the simultaneous supply of individually dosed high-quality amino acids (AM formula blend), the 559 athletes showed a very low rate of infection and few injuries to the tendon-ligament apparatus and minor degenerative changes in the cartilage structures. Substantially higher training continuity was detected in comparison with the competitive athletes who had not received individual micronutrient formulations.

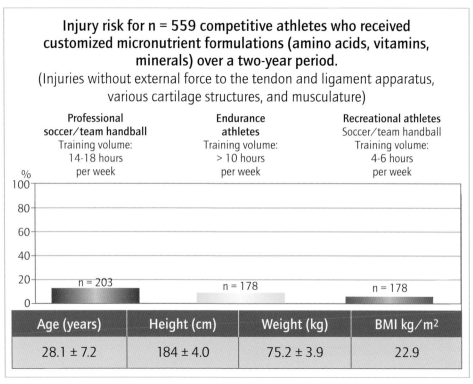

Fig. 4

Status quo of the micronutrient balance in athletes

But not only top competitive athletes are at risk, but rather across the board from recreational athletes to Olympians show noticeable micronutrient supply deficiencies – and the proven benefits of acustomized supplement of these substances. This is shown in the diagrams below along with our test results from various groups.

Assessment of the micronutrient analysis is based on deviation from the respective median and not the concentrations of individual elements. The basis is 9,150 top athletes and 6,434 recreational athletes. Assessment criteria for deviations from the median values:

- Up to − 10% of the median: slight deficiency
- Up to − 20% of the median: definite deficiency
- Up to − 30% of the median: blatant deficiency
- Up to + 20% of the median: requires optimization
- > + 25% of the median: optimal supply

The results from our database show adequateconservation of connective tissue function at > 20% above the respective median value of the micronutrient concentrations.

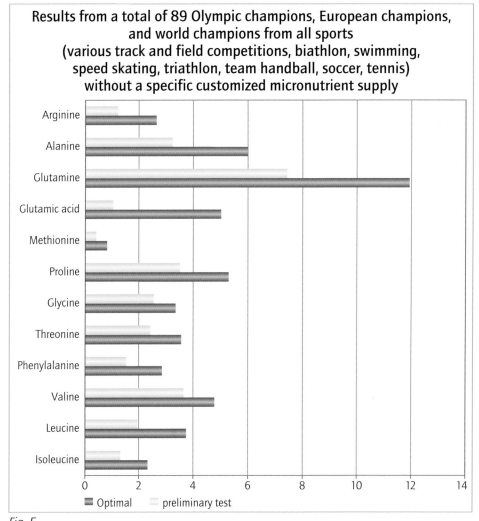

Results from a total of 89 Olympic champions, European champions, and world champions from all sports (various track and field competitions, biathlon, swimming, speed skating, triathlon, team handball, soccer, tennis) without a specific customized micronutrient supply

■ Optimal   ▨ preliminary test

Fig. 5

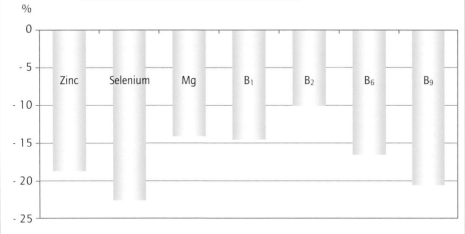

Blatant deficiencies of the intraerythrocytic micronutrient concentration

Measurement of the intracellular micronutrient concentration in 89 top professional athletes without a previous supply of customized micronutrient formulations

Fig. 6

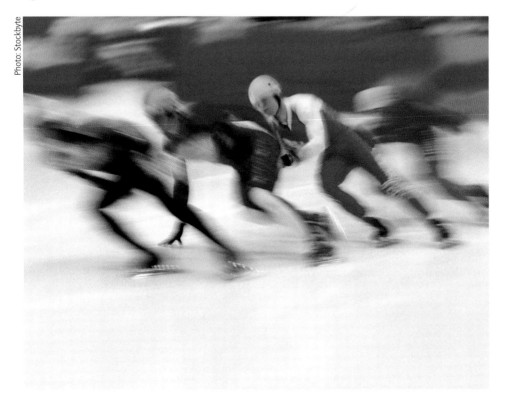

Results from a total of 2,170 competitive athletes with a specific customized micronutrient formulation:

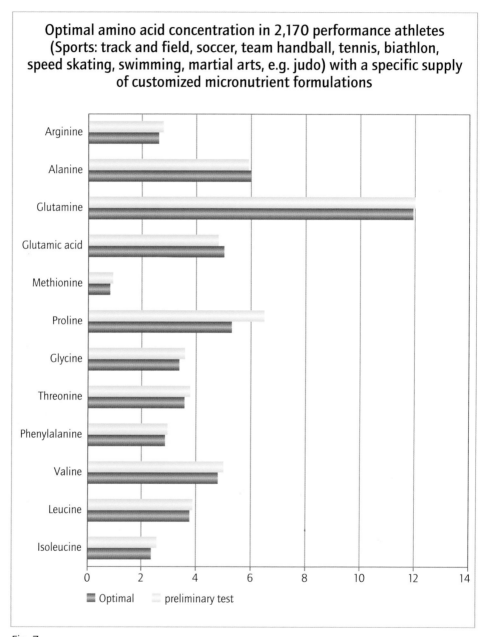

Optimal amino acid concentration in 2,170 performance athletes (Sports: track and field, soccer, team handball, tennis, biathlon, speed skating, swimming, martial arts, e.g. judo) with a specific supply of customized micronutrient formulations

Fig. 7

Optimal development of intraerythrocytic micronutrient concentration with specific customized micronutrient formulations

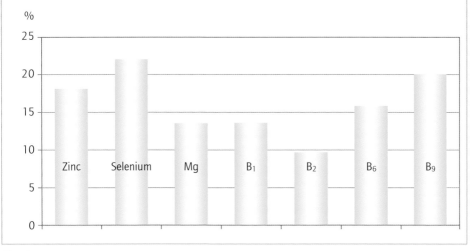

Measurement of intracellular micronutrient concentration in 2,170 competitive athletes after the athletes received customized micronutrient formulations.

Fig. 8

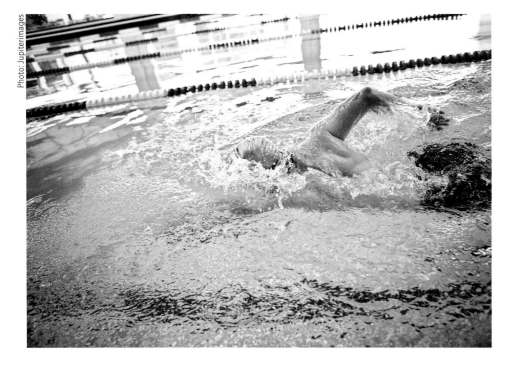

Photo: Jupiterimages

Results from a total of 1,890 competitive athletes without a micronutrient supply:

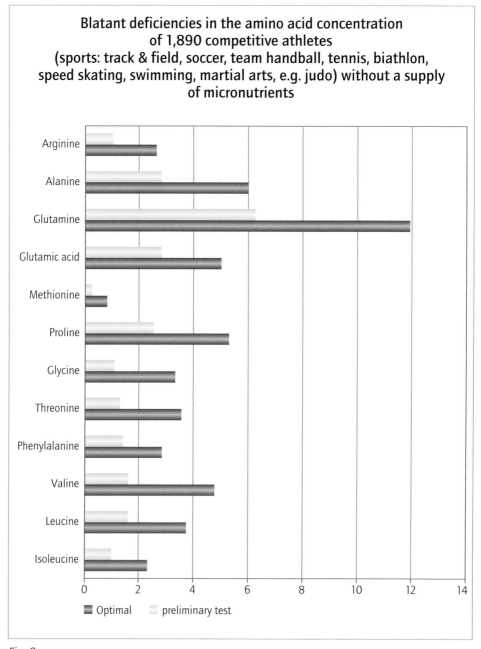

Blatant deficiencies in the amino acid concentration
of 1,890 competitive athletes
(sports: track & field, soccer, team handball, tennis, biathlon,
speed skating, swimming, martial arts, e.g. judo) without a supply
of micronutrients

■ Optimal   ▨ preliminary test

Fig. 9

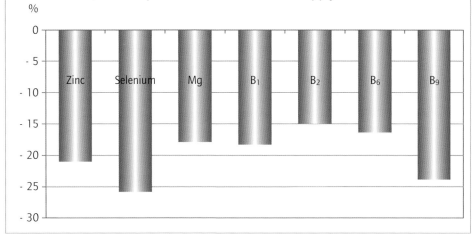

Blatant deficiencies in the forming of the intraerythrocytic micronutrient concentration in 1,890 competitive athletes without a supply of micronutrients

Measurement of the intracellular micronutrient concentration in 1,890 competitive athletes without a supply of micronutrients.

Fig. 10

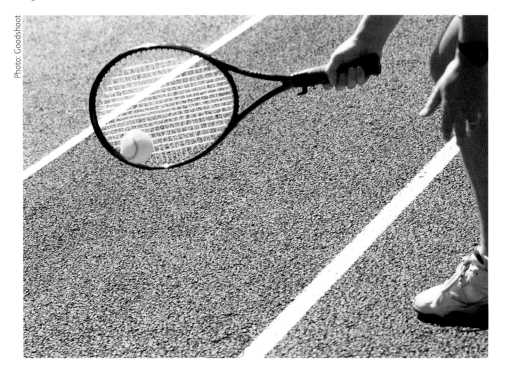

Results from a total of 1,690 recreational competitive athletes who regularly used commercially available nutritional supplements (dosed according to German Nutrition Society guidelines):

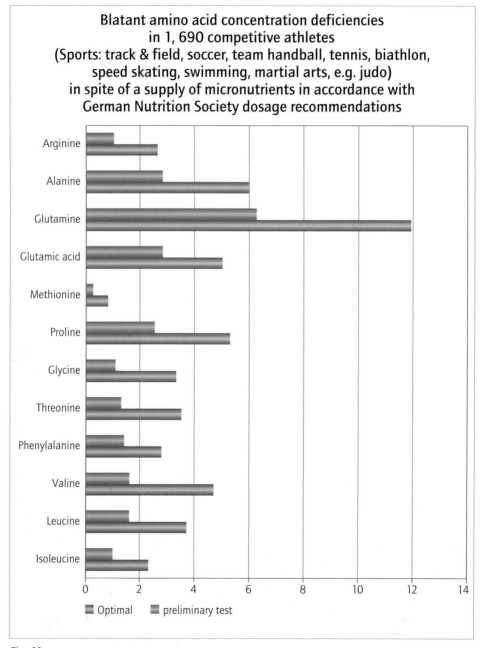

Blatant amino acid concentration deficiencies
in 1, 690 competitive athletes
(Sports: track & field, soccer, team handball, tennis, biathlon,
speed skating, swimming, martial arts, e.g. judo)
in spite of a supply of micronutrients in accordance with
German Nutrition Society dosage recommendations

Fig. 11

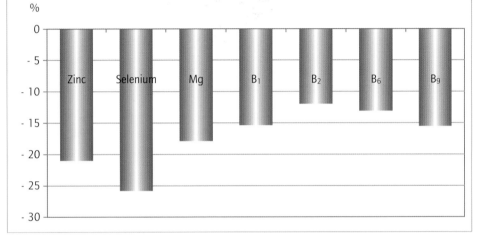

**Blatant deficiencies in the forming of the intraerythrocytic
micronutrient concentrationin spite of a supply of micronutrients
in accordance with German Nutrition Society
dosage recommendations**

Intracellular micronutrient concentration deficiencies in 1,690
competitive athletes in spite of a supply of micronutrients

Fig. 12

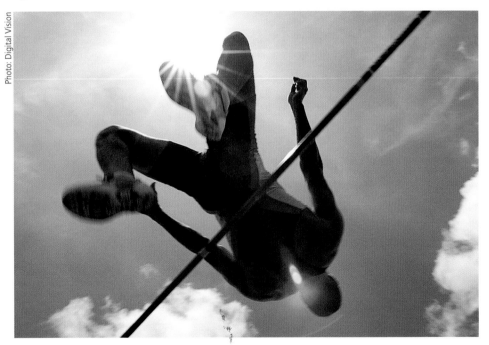

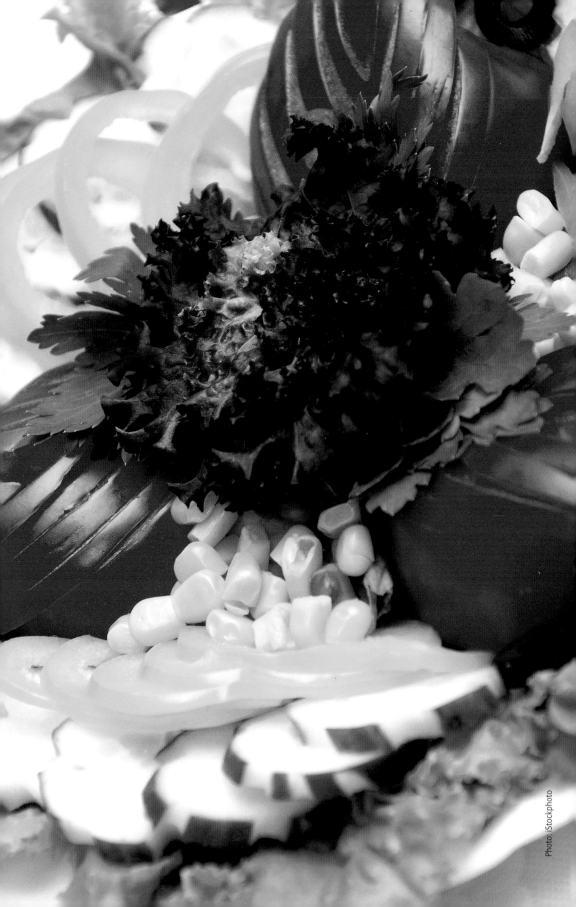

2 You are what you eat – nutritional physiological aspects

2.1 About the necessity of supplying athletes with micronutrients

Full of life, fit and productive as long as possible – that is what trainers and players wish for. Everyone knows about the close relationship between nutrition, immune system and performance. Some may wonder why they don't feel so great and aren't very productive, in spite of a balanced diet. In this chapter we will present some correlations that may be somewhat surprising and make a case for the necessary and specific supply of micronutrients.

The engine won't run without gas

The maintenance of vital functions absolutely requires a sufficient supply of minerals and trace elements. In particular zinc, selenium, magnesium and all of the B-vitamins (i. e. B_1, B_2, B_6, B_9, B_{12}) play an essential part in a number of physiological processes of cell metabolism, cell division, stability, energy metabolism and immune response. More recent findings show higher micronutrient requirements of amino acids, which are needed for the stabilization and development of many connective tissue structures (ligaments, tendons, cartilage) during phases of intensive training and competition. Future long-term tests done with MRT imaging (magnetic resonance imaging) will substantiate this.

Based on our new findings, micronutrient deficiencies can lead to premature degeneration of connective tissue structures and increase the risk of injuryin the long-term. Particularly in recreational, competitive and top competitive athletes, deficiencies as well as a suboptimal supply can affect the immune system, which provides a significant foundation for the continuity of training and competing.

Our experiences in the care recreational and competitive athletes, show that significant deficiencies in the cellular micronutrient supply exist in nearly all areas, which has lead to a variety of medical conditions in the athletes.

Personal studies (incl. clinical studies) and projects during recent years prove that even with a balanced diet (based on criteria of the German Nutrition Society) a serious micronutrient deficiency can be detected in the cell, that cannot be sufficiently corrected without a specific supply of micronutrients. Special reference should be made to the specific cellular measuring and diagnostics of these deficiencies. There are very few laboratories in Europe that conduct cellular analyses and have access to an adequate databank with athletes.

Cellular blood tests reveal deficiencies

According to the DGE's most recent nutrition report and statements by renowned nutrition scientists, sports scientists and sports medicine specialists, an additional supply of micronutrients for athletes is not necessary as long as they have a balanced diet (except for fluoride, iodine and folic acid; the insufficient supply beyond the standard diet in Germany is well-known).

Our experiences while caring for recreational and competitive athletes were quite different.

Their nutrition log, which was analyzed with the help of nutrition scientists, did in fact not lead to the conclusion that the athletes who had been examined had any deficiencies in their micronutrient supply. However, the cellular blood tests showed a significant under-supply. This was accompanied by various ailments (discomfort in the tendon-ligament apparatus, in various cartilage structures, decreased performance, increased fatigue, lack of progress in training).

Accurate micronutrient diagnostics are essential – micronutrient deficiencies often remain undiagnosed

If measured at all, vitamins and trace elements are usually measured in the blood but not in the cell. Blood serum tests are not valid with respect to actual supply of micronutrients to the cell. A drop in the levels is only perceptible when characteristic deficiency symptoms or even tissue or organ damage occurs. But a latent under-supply may have been in existence for an extended period of time without any obvious acute health problems.

Blood is the mode of transportation. The concentration of minerals, trace elements and other micronutrients depends strongly on the recent and present ingestion of these substances, e.g. through nourishment.

Routine blood tests are done on the serum level where red and white blood cells are no longer present. The level readings are thus extracellular (extracellular = existing outside the cell; opposite = intracellular). Elements with a predominantly intracellular concentration, such as potassium, magnesium, zinc, and the B-vitamins (B_1, B_2, B_6, B_9) cannot be detected. Element determinations in blood serum thus do not offer reliable conclusions with respect to mineral, vitamin and trace element balance.

Important biochemical effect mechanisms of elements occur primarlily on the cellular level. The determination of element concentrations from serum can therefore not provide information about celllular processes.

The exchange between extra and intracellular space is regulated through complex autologous mechanisms. The concentration of essential elements in the serum is kept as constant as possible. Autologous reserves are mobilized to maintain the serum level if the micronutrient supply (vitamins, minerals etc.) is insufficient to do so. That is why deficiencies in the serum are most often not detected or only very late. By 9.150 competitive and 6.434 recreational athletes no deficiencies were detected on the serum level, but definite deficiencies were detected on the cellular level. When deficiencies exist on the serum level, deficiencies in the cell are detectable considerably sooner.

Problems may have existed for a long time but their cause cannot be established through routine blood tests: decreased concentration ability, increased fatigue, muscle tension and all the way to allergic reactions to pollen, are just some of the complex symptoms.

Even if there are no actual ailments, the goal should be notto use up one's individual resources. According to our initial research findings, the degeneration of many connective tissue structures (tendons, ligaments, cartilage) will only surface after months, if not years. This can be prevented with the timely replenishing of cellular stores (see pg. 107-108).

2.2 Brief digression on the components of blood

Blood is, for all intents and purposes, the body's liquid transportation tissue, or rather the assistant to the circulatory system. Its job is to provide a supply of the things that are vital to each cell, like fuel from nutrition, oxygen, vitamins, hormones, and warmth, and then to eliminate metabolic waste products as well as warmth from each cell.

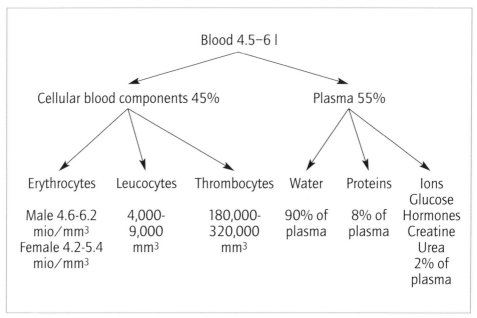

Fig. 13

The total volume of circulating blood in a human body is approximately 8% of the total body weight. Thus a person weighing 176 lbs. has a blood volume of approximately 1.69 gallons. Blood consists of liquid and solid components: liquid components are referred to as blood plasma, and solid components are referred to as blood corpuscle.

Blood plasma

Blood plasma is a clear liquid. It consists of 93% water and contains substances such as salt, carbohydrates, lipids and proteins. The white blood cells (leukocytes) are the body's defense mechanism. They combat bacteria, viruses, fungi and parasites that enter the body through skin injuries, respiration or digestion. Red blood cells (erythrocytes), which make up approximately 45% of the total volume, transport oxygen or rather carbon dioxide and contain the red blood pigment (hemoglobin). During the initial years, all of our blood tests were measured in the erythrocytes (intraerythrocytic) as well as the serum. Today micronutrient concentrations are measured exclusively in the red blood cells since routine serum tests verifiably are of no informational value.

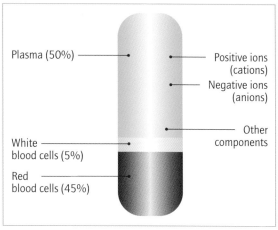

Blood cells

In addition to the blood's liquid (plasma) there are also different blood cells. All of them, with the exception of lymphocytes, which also form in the lymphatic organs, are

Fig. 14

formed in the red bone marrow (medulla ossium rubra). After a certain maturing period they are released into the blood. Their percentage within the blood varies greatly.

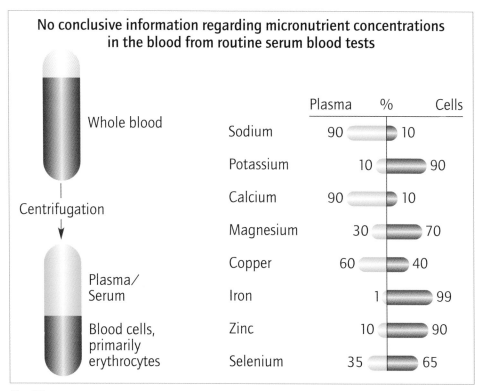

No conclusive information regarding micronutrient concentrations in the blood from routine serum blood tests

	Plasma	%	Cells
Sodium	90		10
Potassium	10		90
Calcium	90		10
Magnesium	30		70
Copper	60		40
Iron	1		99
Zinc	10		90
Selenium	35		65

Fig. 15

Red blood cells (erythrocytes) are viable for approximately three months. Then they are replaced. A male has approximately 5 million erythrocytes within one cubic millimeter; a female has approximately 4.5 million. Their primary function is to transport oxygen from the pulmonary alveoli to the organs, as well as the transport of carbon dioxide from the tissue back to the to the alveoli.

White blood cells (leukocytes) are present in the blood at a rate of 5,000 to 6,000 per cubic milliliter. The number of different white blood cells present at any given time varies during the course of one's life and during the course of illnesses. Leukocytes include lymphocytes, granulocytes, monocytes that can be indentified in a differential blood count. Leukocytes can live anywhere from a few hours to several years.

Platelets (thrombocytes) occur at a rate of 150.000 to 350.000 per cubic milliliter. They play a very important role in the clotting process because they seal the vascular walls when an injury occurs. The thrombocytes' life span is 5 to 10 days.

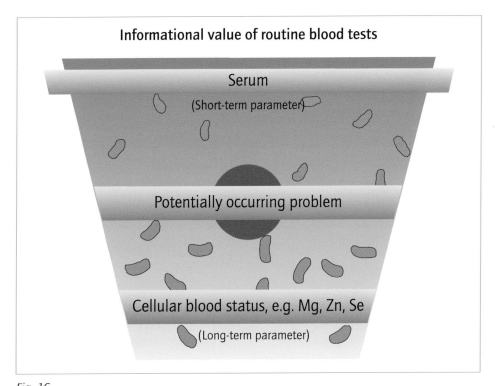

Fig. 16

Important information

All possible autologous resources, particularly from the cellular level, are mobilized to retain important micronutrients on the serum level. That is why deficiencies on the serum level are detected late or not at all.

The following illustrations show significant individual micronutrient concentration deficiencies in cellular blood tests (lower than the reference range) of 508 test subjects, even though serum levels are almost exclusively within the reference range (normal range).

Example: frequency distribution (%) of serum and intracellular blood counts (in erythrocytes) in 508 subjects (Wienecke, 2007)

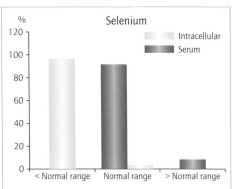
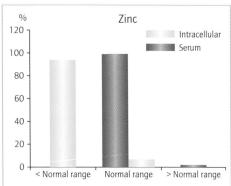
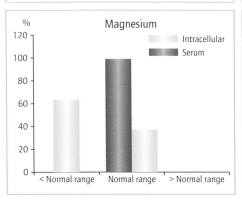
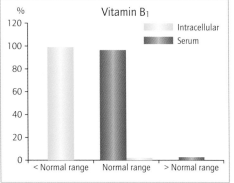

Fig. 17

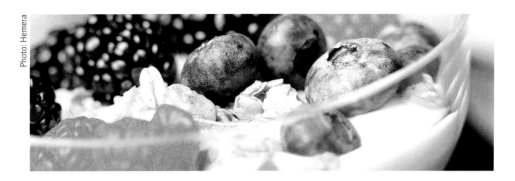

Photo: Hemera

Important information

To conduct a reliable interpretation of the micronutrient results, the designation as a percent deviation from the median of the collective norm (6,434 recreational and 9,150 top athletes) must be taken into account when interpreting the cellular micronutrient analysis.

Assessment of the micronutrient analysis is based on deviation from the respective median and not the concentrations of individual elements. The basis for this analysis are 9,150 top athletes and 6,434 recreational athletes. Assessment criteria for deviations from the median values:

- Up to – 10% of the median: slight deficiency
- Up to – 20% of the median: definite deficiency
- Up to – 30% of the median: blatant deficiency
- Up to + 20% of the median: requires optimization
- > + 25% of the median: optimal supply

The results from our database show adequate conservation of connective tissue function at > 20% above the respective median value of the micronutrient concentrations.

2.3   Causes for increased micronutrient deficiencies in athletes in spite of a balanced diet

Latest findings confirm significant loss of micronutrients due to the greenhouse effect

American biologists can explain why we can detect an increasing deficiency in the cellular micronutrient balance in spite of a balanced diet: The increase in CO_2 emissions seems to have a not insignificant impact on the decrease of micronutrient concentrations in today's food. The content of substances specified word-wide appears to be outdated.

Today, one can assume that there is a considerable decrease in substance of content in foods. If deficiencies on this scale were measured during an experiment in the course of six months, the actual losses during the past decades are much greater. This is said to be one of the main reasons why especially people who actively engage in sports are unable to achieve a sufficient micronutrient supply in spite of a balanced diet. Next to the massive impact of micronutrient deficiencies due to the greenhouse effect shown below, there are additional confounding factors, such as incorrect preparation and losses during storage.

Background information

The American biologist Iraki Loladze of Princeton University, New Jersey, had already reported on initial testing in 2002, and determined that the increase in CO_2 emissions even during the past decades has lead to a definite reduction in substance of content. There is no other explanation for the results from our clinical study with 100 women and 76 students who had a very health-conscious diet (see pg. 40-51). His research up to 2002 specifies essentially two processes:

1. Increased CO_2 emissions increases plant growth and thus crop yields which, however, takes place at the expense of valuable substance of content (trace elements, other micronutrients).

2. The elevated CO_2 levelslimit plants' transpiration. Because less water evaporates through the leaves, less water is also absorbed from the ground. This diminished water supply leads to the decreased availability of iron, magnesium and zinc from the ground.

A likely conclusion would be that today there is at least a 30% to 40% reduction in substance of content in food!

(Wienecke, 2005)

In a pilot project at the Technical University Braunschweig, Germany, scientists simulated the greenhouse effect in the year 2050. The results showed a definite reduction of micronutrients (zinc, selenium etc., and also protein concentrations) in the plants that were being tested (with the exception of calcium). Plants will grow more quickly but will contain considerably fewer micronutrients.

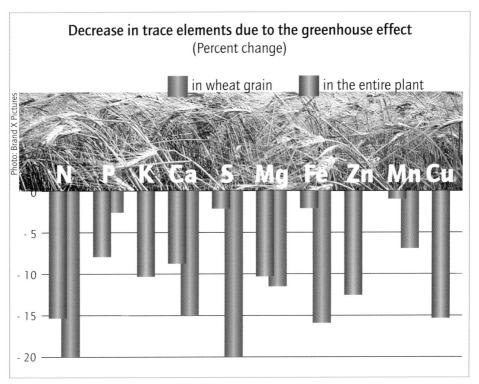

Fig. 18: During the experiment wheat plants in a greenhouse received twice as much CO_2 as in open land (from "Trends of Ecology & Evolution", 2002).

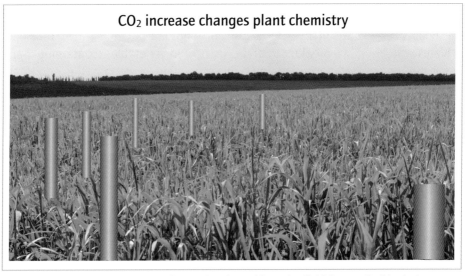

Fig. 19: CO_2 test area (simulation): CO_2 is released into the field from cylindrical pipes.

In the fall of 2008, one of the most renowned television shows on the German TV-channel *ZDF*, "Abenteuer Wissen", showed the TU Braunschweig's research results in a test field.

2.4 For many athletes a healthy diet is an unattainable optimum

Everyone senses the close relationship between nutrition and performance. By now there are countless books that deal with this topic more or less objectively. We will therefore not list any details but rather focus on good nutrition in general (detailed tips, see pg. 213-238) and on a targeted qualitative and quantitative supplementary micronutrient supply in particular, which is the subject of much controversy among sports medicine specialists and nutrition scientists.

Expedient only in combinations

Based on the results listed thus far one could get the impression that athletes depend on an additional supply of micronutrients and that a good diet has far less impact on the micronutrient balance than previously thought.

Far from it! It is true that there is an urgent need for a specific customized micronutrient formulation (not according to the shotgun approach and in the believe that "a lot helps a lot"). But our longtime research shows that only athletes who also have a balanced diet of fruits and vegetables (containing many as of yet unexplored secondary nutrients) are able to absorb the additional micronutrients.

Anyone who thinks he can ease a guilty conscience with a regular supply of vitamins, minerals and trace elements – along the lines of eating fast food and take pills – has not really understood the problem. Our research clearly shows that recreational or top competitive athletes are not able to meet their personal requirements of cellular micronutrients in spite of a good diet. You should therefore pay attention to your athletes' diet and a qualitatively sensible supplement.

2.5 Physical exertion in sports increases micronutrient requirements

Initial findings from preliminary tests

In the course of a screening campaign with the Bertelsmann Foundation of 310 subjects with various ailments, who were involved in practically no athletics, we were unable to detect any deficiencies on the serum level while significant deficiencies were detected on the cellular level (see illustration). The diet of this subject group was consistent with that of the general population, meaning it was not particularly good.

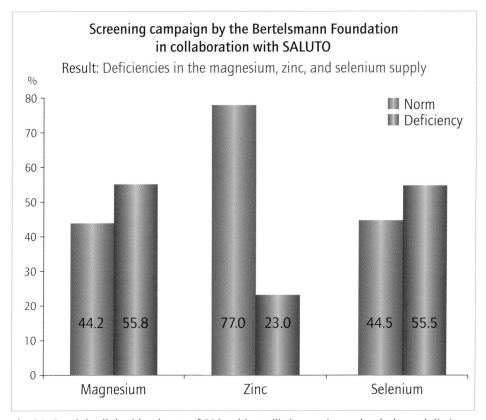

Fig. 20: Special cellular blood tests of 310 subjects (little exercise and unbalanced diet)

During various research projects we specifically looked into the questions of how physical exertion in sports can impact micronutrient deficiency and whether or not an optimal diet can combat deficiencies in the micronutrient balance. Overall we measured the micronutrient balance on a cellular level of 715 people who had completed an individual 40-minute cardio workout three times a week. In addition nutrition scientists did three one-week nutritional analyses,which determined that compared to the general population, this particular group of people had a good diet.

However, in the Bertelsmann Foundation screening campaign the cellular deficiencies increased further in comparison to the inactive group (see Fig. 21).

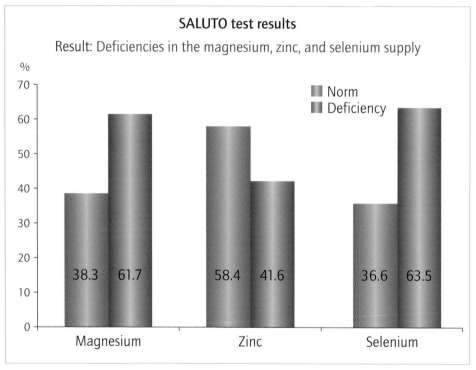

Fig. 21: Status quo of 715 physically active subjects (3 x 40 minutes per week moderate endurance training). Balanced diet in accordance with German Nutrition Society guidelines

Optimal nutrition cannot meet micronutrient requirements even in recreational athletes – newest findings

A pilot project with students produced astonishing results on this issue. For this purpose we took care of 76 students at an all-day school, morning, afternoon and evening, for a period of four months, with the aid of a nutritionist. In biology class the students learned about the significance of nutrition and the theoretical background information. Together the students planned their breakfast in the mornings and received practical support. Three times a week, during the school day, the students completed a 40-minute endurance workout with individual pulse rate guidelines under the direction of a certified sports scientist.

The students' diet revealed extremely positive results. The students met more than 85% of the nutrition guidelines propagated by the German Nutrition Society. The students also met these guidelines in the area of good fats (high-grade omega 3 fatty acids).

Although the students had a very good diet at the all-day school during the research period with the help of a nutritionist, the cellular micronutrient stores were clearly reduced due to the active moderate 40-minute endurance workout three times a week (see Fig 23). Ailments such as pollen allergies increased significantly. Only the decrease in cellular zinc and magnesium stores is listed here as an example.

Results of this pilot study

These results (see Fig 22-23) clearly demonstrate the need for specific supplements in spite of a balanced diet. Please take into account that the majority of all students does not have a balanced diet, and their micronutrient balance therefore shows much more serious deficiencies.

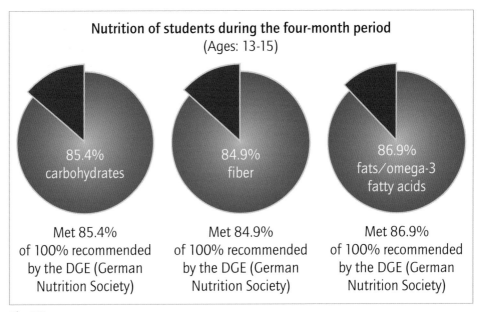

Nutrition of students during the four-month period
(Ages: 13-15)

85.4% carbohydrates

84.9% fiber

86.9% fats/omega-3 fatty acids

Met 85.4% of 100% recommended by the DGE (German Nutrition Society)

Met 84.9% of 100% recommended by the DGE (German Nutrition Society)

Met 86.9% of 100% recommended by the DGE (German Nutrition Society)

Fig. 22

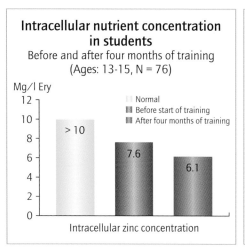

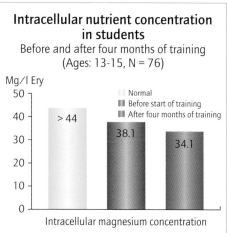

Fig. 23

First clinical study
with 100 women eating a good diet, at SALUTO Institute

The clinical study was initiated and conducted by SALUTO and was conducted by IFAT (Institute for Applied Telemedicine) at the Heart and Diabetes Center along with additional physicians, natural and nutrition scientists, and SALUTO biologists. The goal of this placebo-controlled, randomized, double blind nutrition study was to demonstrate the need for supplementation with minerals, trace elements and vitamins in healthy adult female subjects with recommended physical or rather athletic activity and a healthy diet by means of a specific supply of these substances, and their effects on the cellular stores and the endurance capacity.

Preliminary testing (screening) was done before the study began. During this screening all of the subjects completed a nutrition analysis to make sure that only subjects with a "balanced diet" as per the Nutrition Society, would be included in the study.

The 100 subjects included in the study were randomly distributed between the verum group (VG) and the placebo group (PG) (50 subjects per group). They took a daily combination of a commercial Taxofit assortment of vitamins, minerals and trace elements over a four-month period. The dosage of the ingested micronutrients was in accordance with nutritional supplement criteria (i.a. 15 mg zinc, 50 µg, 2 x 250 mg of magnesium, and 800 µg of folic acid) in a specially developed formulation. No vitamin B_1 and B_2 was given.

Clinical study Basis is N = 100 women		
	Verum	Placebo
Age	45.6	45.8
Weight (kg)	66.0	69.2
BMI	24.1	24.7
Resting heart rate	75.8	78.4
Blood pressure	130/84	130/85

Fig. 24

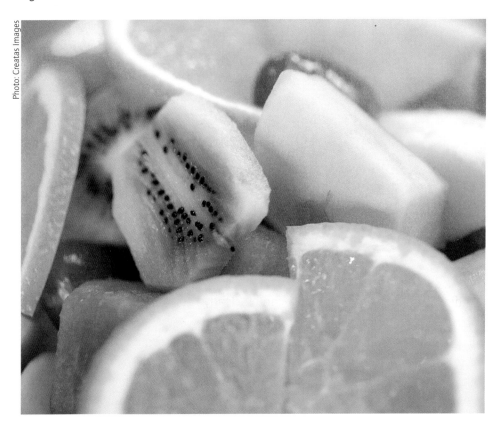

Photo: Creatas Images

While taking the test supplements the subjects participated in a four-month long exercise program (cardio-pulmonary training) three times a week for 40 minutes. Each participant exercised according to specified individual intensity levels that had been determined by us based on exercise stress tests. Monitoring was done with the Polar team system, which documented the individual training units via heart rate.

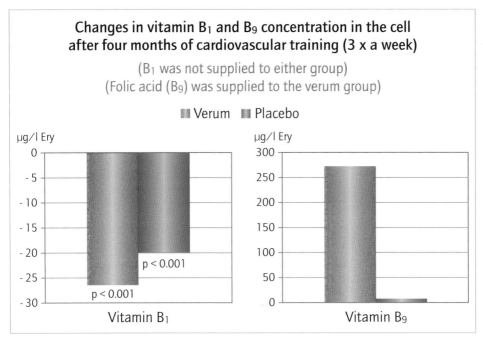

Fig. 25

The results

Micronutrient requirements could not be met in spite of a good diet along with moderate endurance training three times a week for 40 minutes. Cellular micronutrient stores clearly decreased (see Fig 25). Placebo and verum comparison showed significant differences. Contrary to doctrine in sports science, sports medicine and nutrition science, it can be clearly shown that a targeted supply of micronutrients (trace elements, minerals) is necessary for the individual engaging in athletic activity. Shown here by example, the cellular B_1 concentration (this was not supplied in verum vs. placebo) and B_9 (folic acid).

Conclusion: The "status quo" of the micronutrient balance can only be accurately measured with the aid of special cellular blood tests.

Diagnostics matter

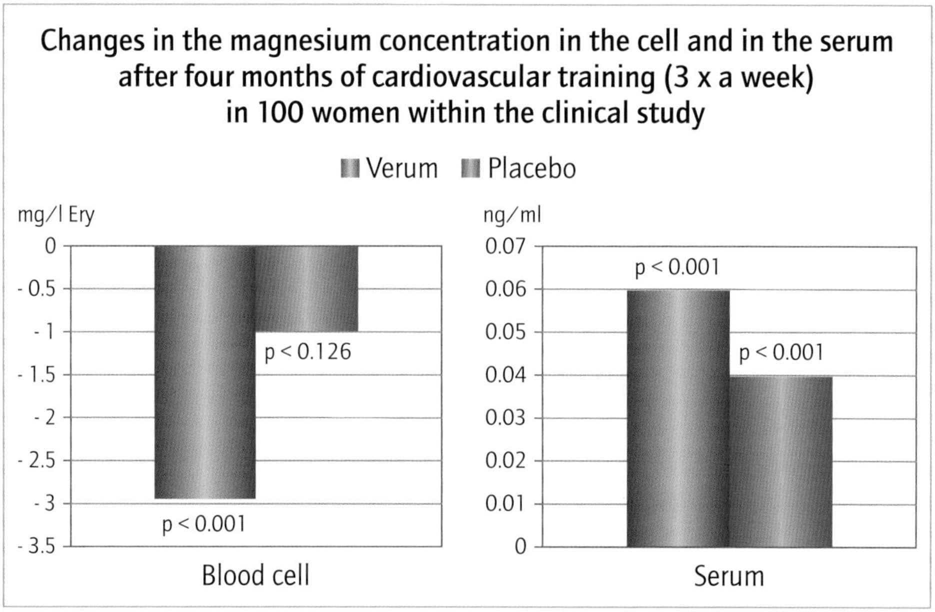

Fig. 26

Cardiovascular parameter before and after four months
Clinical study (N = 100 female test subjects)

	Verum		Placebo	
	T_1	T_2	T_1	T_2
Weight	66.0	65.2	69.2	67.8
BMI	24.1	23.8	24.7	24.6
Heart rate	75.8	71.1	78.4	73.0
Blood pressure	130/84	127/82	130/85	127/81
Cholesterol	199.3	188.3	199.0	187.4
HDL	62.2	64.9	67.1	67.5
LDL	113.6	97.0	115.3	100.9
Triglycerides	82.8	97.5	83.2	94.2

Fig. 27

As an additional example of optimal diagnostics we can illustrate the development of the cellular magnesium concentration in our clinical study with 100 women eating a good diet. While the cellular magnesium concentration clearly decreased in the verum as well as the placebo group, a statistically significant increase could be seen on the serum level, which will however lead to a misinterpretation of the results.

Photo: Stockbyte

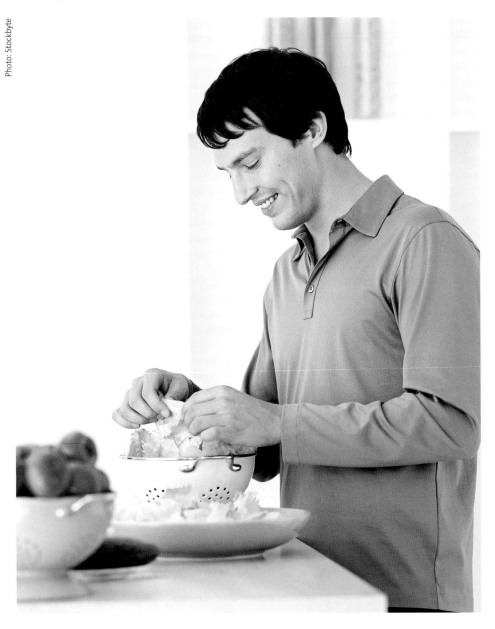

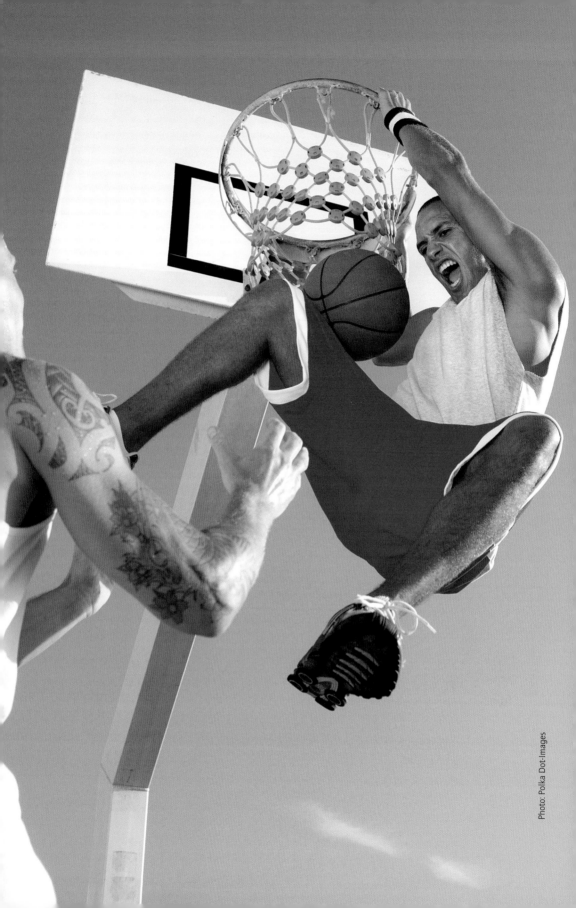

3 Composition of body tissue essential to athletic performance

3.1 Strong tissue structures protect from injuries and assure athletic success

Brief characterization of different connective tissue structures

Tissue refers to cells performing a common function that have formed united structures: They are the building material for the organs and organ systems of the human body and have specific functions.

There are different types of tissue:

- Muscle tissue, which facilitates movement, is composed of many cells that are fused together, the muscle fibers with their elastic components. Here we differentiate between *smooth* and *striated* muscle tissue.

- Connective and supporting tissue, consisting of cartilage and bone cells, supports the body. It holds the body's organs, fills the gaps in between and stores fat, thereby providing pressure-resistant cushioning.

- The epithelium is once more differentiated, depending on the predominant function. We differentiate between *sensory epithelia* (structure of sensory organs), *tubular epithelia* (secretion and reabsorption) and *glandular epithelia* (secretion production).

- The brain and spinal cord are made up of nerve tissue. It provides nourishment and support for nerve cells and insulates the individual nerve fibers.

Connective and supporting tissue

Connective and supporting tissue consists of very varied macroporous cell structures. These include on the one hand the parts of the skeleton such as bones, cartilage, ligaments and tendons; on the other hand the reticular weave that connects organs and organ parts and holds them in place.

Although they are very different on the outside, they share a common origin and therefore are closely connected. That is to say they originate from an embryonic connective tissue *(mesenchyme)*. Mesenchyme cells form a loose, spongy cell structure whose gaps are filled with a liquid substance (matrix). This substance contains dissolved salts and proteins. Cells within the embryonic connective tissue can divide and separate from their structure. This creates large scavenger cells *(macrophages)*. Contrary to connective and supporting tissue, muscle, nerve and epithelia tissue consists mostly of cellular structures.

The involvement of cells and matrix in the development of connective tissue and supporting tissue structures varies. The more prominent the supporting function, the lower the metabolic function, and vice-versa.

An optimal micronutrient supply stabilizes the structure of taut connective tissue

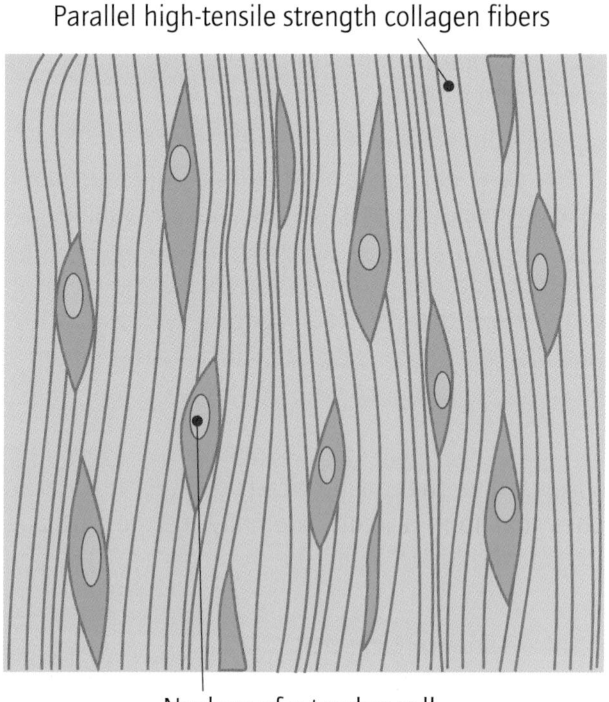

Parallel high-tensile strength collagen fibers

Nucleus of a tendon cell

Fig. 28

Next to connective tissue, fat tissue, cartilage and bone are part of the main supporting tissues.

3.2 Cartilage

Cartilage tissue occurs primarily in the skeleton and the air passages. It is firm but elastic when bent or pushed.

This is due to the strong intercellular matter that forms the cartilage tissue together with the cartilage cells. *Hyalinecartilage, fibro cartilage* and *elastic cartilage* can be differentiated by the different ratios between intercellular matter and cells.

Cartilage cells *(chondrocytes)* usually have a rounded appearance with an equally round nucleus. They can be found in small chondrocyte groups where they are generally arranged in columns or rows. Cartilage cells are high in water, fat and glycogen.

The intercellular matter (matrix) consists of up to 70% water; in addition collagen fiber bundles, protein and elastin are embedded.

In an adult it is free of blood vessels and its nutrient supply occurs through the surrounding tissue such as the *perichondrium*, or via the joint fluid *(synovia)*. The nutrient supply decreases over the course of life, which can lead to attrition of the joints (osteoarthritis).

Hyaline cartilage

Hyaline cartilage has a milky-blue colorand appears transparent and glass-like. It can absorb strong pressure. That is why it can be found as a smoothing surface on the ends of bones that form a joint. Externally hyaline cartilage is encased by *perichondrium* that merges directly into the cartilage.

The pressure resistant intercellular matter (matrix) contains collagen fibrillae and non-collagen protein matter. Cells with high water content, surrounded by a capsule, are located in so-called cartilage *cavities*. They are separated from the matrix by a lacuna and together with the shell, or rather capsule that surrounds them they form a *chondron* (cartilage that functionally belongs together).

During the embryonic stage hyaline cartilage forms the skeletal bones, which gradually change to bone tissue. It also facilitates continued growth in height up to adult seize via the existing physical cartilage at the point of transition from the epiphysis to the diaphysis. Degenerative processes can occur in old age due to the decrease in nutrients; furthermore early calcium deposits in hyaline cartilage must be monitored.

Occurrence of hyaline cartilage: Rib cartilage, joint cartilage, epiphysial cartilage, nasal septum (partially), and laryngeal skeleton.

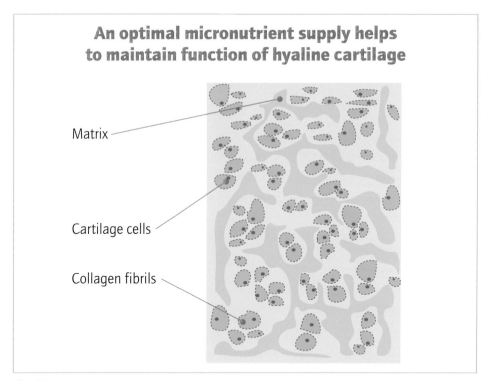

Fig. 29

Fibro cartilage

Compared to hyaline cartilage, fibro cartilage or rather connective tissue cartilage contains much more collagen fibers. They form a meshwork of strong overlapping

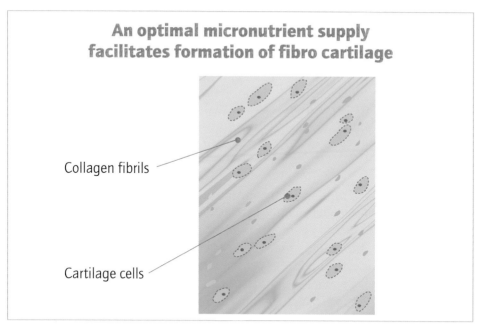

Fig. 30

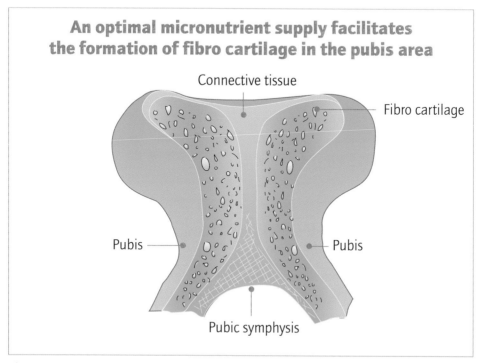

Fig. 31

fibrillae (small fibers). Scattered in between are individual cartilage cells which, compared to hyaline and elastic cartilage, are fewer in number.

Fibro cartilage has a lot of tensile strength and can be found anywhere where pressure is placed on ligaments or tendons. It can therefore be found in parts of the intervertebral disks (disci intervertebrales), but also in menisci, flexible disks (disci articulares), and in the pubic symphysis.

Elastic cartilage

Contrary to the bluish hyaline cartilage, elastic cartilage has a yellowish color. Its intercellular matter (matrix) contains a lot of elastic fiber meshwork and fewer collagen fibers. They are arranged net-like around the cartilage cells (chondrocytes) and extend into the perichondrium. This is what gives the elastic cartilage its flexibility and elasticity. Elastic cartilage can be found, among others, in the epiglottis, the eustachian tube (tuba auditiva), and the auricle.

Cartilage nourishment

- Mature cartilage contains either blood or lymph vessels. Vessels are not really expedient in a tissue that primarily serves the absorption of impact, compressive and tractive force. Exceptions: embryonic hyaline cartilage and areas of hyaline cartilage ossification.

- The supply of nutrients and respiratory gas to the cartilage cells occurs through hyaline and elastic cartilage, generally by diffusion from the perichondrium, except for hyaline cartilage joints, which are supplied directly via the synovia.

- Fibro cartilage that lacks a perichondrium receives its supply from the adjacent connective tissue, the hyaline cartilage or bone.

- Thus cartilage is by nature a tissue with relatively slow metabolic activity, a so-called *bradythrophic* tissue.

- Due to the fact that supply paths automatically get longer, particularly because of the interstitial growth, any volume expansion of cartilage tissue has metabolism-relatedlimits.

Conclusion: Additionally it is not unusual for intensive training and resulting serious micronutrient deficiencies to further impede the metabolic matrix (see pg. 82-85). Amino acids (i.a. methionine, proline, arginine, cysteine) that are jointly responsible for connective tissue development, are increasingly drawn on for catabolic purposes, so that they are not sufficiently available for the stabilization or rather the development of additional connective tissue structures (i.a. cartilage). As a result there is the potential for long-term incrustation and demasking of collagen fibers, but also premature degenerative deformation. Our experiences in recent years while caring for athletes show that a targeted micronutrient therapy can provide optimal protection through prevention (see pg. 107-108).

3.3 Muscle tissue

Muscles are composed of muscle cells which have the ability to contract longitudinally with nerve stimulation. Embedded in the muscle cells are small contractile protein threads (so called *myofibrils*). They contract when stimulated, and return to their original shape when stimulus ceases. All muscle tissue also contains connective tissue, whose purpose is to connect the muscle cells. In addition the connective tissue transmits the muscle contraction to the surrounding area. The most important property of muscle tissue, the ability to contract, allows the bones to move against each other within the skeletal system.

Muscle fiber or muscle cells are differentiated by their cell structure and according to their function as:

• smooth muscle

• striated muscle, and

• heartmuscle.

Striated muscle is composed of various tissues: Striated muscle fibers make up the bulk. They form the entire skeletal musculature that facilitates movement and is involved in muscle reflex. Its function is to move the skeletal bones against each other. These arbitrary movements are initiated by the cerebral cortex and reach the muscles via nerve tracts in the spinal cord (medulla spinalis) and motor nerves. Skeletal muscles can also be found to a small extent in the Internal organs of the head and throat, the tongue (lingua), the throat (pharynx) and the esophagus.

Multiple muscle fibers are combined into bundles and muscles via connective tissue fibers. The muscle fibers themselves are multinuclear, cylinder-shaped cylindrical cells that can get up to 12 cm long and up to 100 μ thick (1 mm = 1000 μm). Their striations stem from the myofibrils that are located in the cells.

The cells with their nuclei lie directly below the surface, specifically with their longitudinal axis pointed in the direction of the fibers. Under a microscope one can see alternately double and single-refracting sections. Here we can distinguish that the myofibrils consist of thick and thin myosin filaments. Thicker filaments relate to the double-refractive sections, and thinner ones to the single-refractive sections.

Muscle structure – principal components

In a narrower sense only the muscle fibers can contract and be built up through workload or sports.

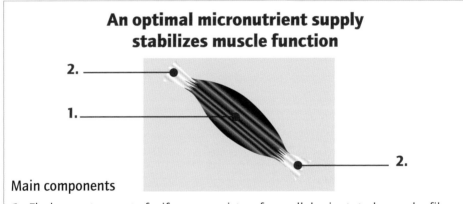

Main components

1. Fleshy center part, fusiform; consists of parallel-orientated muscle fibers bundled into strands.

2. Connective tissue ligaments that connect the ends of muscle tissue to the bone (not present in the ring muscles of the lips or the dermal muscles); they can be very short, but also very long (e.g. finger and toe flexors and extensors).

Fig. 32

Muscle structure –fine structure

1. The muscle's smallest functional unit capable of contracting is the *muscle fibril*, consisting of thin actin filaments alternating with thicker myosin filaments. During contraction the muscle shortens because the actin and myosin filaments telescope.

2. The muscle fibrils are arranged in muscle fibers, meaning thousands of muscle cells with a thin membrane, each housing a nucleus and various structures for production of energy such as the mitochondria. This is where the nerve fibers begin to trigger the muscle contraction.

3. The muscle fibers in turn are combined into bundles, each one encased in a connective tissue membrane; these fiber bundles can be seen with the naked eye when cutting a piece of meat.

4. All bundles combined form the muscle.

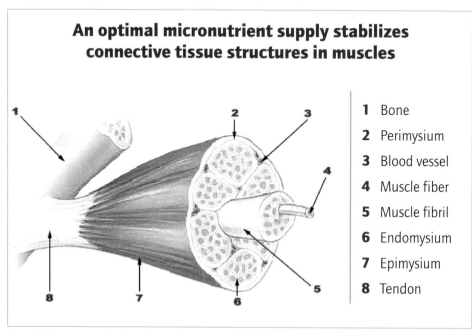

An optimal micronutrient supply stabilizes connective tissue structures in muscles

1 Bone
2 Perimysium
3 Blood vessel
4 Muscle fiber
5 Muscle fibril
6 Endomysium
7 Epimysium
8 Tendon

Fig. 33: Structure of striated muscle

Characteristics of muscles

Skeletal muscles possess four basic characteristics:

- *Contractibility:* The ability to actively contract in response to nerve stimuli or out of reflex.

- *Excitability:* The ability to react to an electric impulse and to transmit that impulse.

- *Flexibility:* The ability to elongate beyond its length in a relaxed state.

- *Elasticity:* The ability to return to its relaxed state after stretching or contracting.

3.4 Tendons and ligaments

Auxiliary organs of the skeletal muscles include tendons, muscle fascia, tendon sheaths, bursa, sesamoid bones, and sesamoid cartilage.

- Tendons transfer muscular pull to the bone. They run into the bone's collagen fibers at the muscle origin (origo) and the muscle insertion (insertio). Tendons consist of collagen fiber bundles with great tensile strength and gather the ends of the muscle fiber bundles into tough rope-like structures. The muscle origin is formed by short tendons such as can be seen in the large pectoral muscle (pectoralis major). The tendons of the hand and foot muscles are comparatively small and long. Tendons with a laminar structure (aponeurosis) occur on oblique abdominal muscles.

- Additional distinctive features are that there are flexor and extensor tendons. Flexor tendons change direction by wrapping around a bone and respond to pressure on the side that faces the bone. An example for this is the tendon origin of the long calf muscle (peroneus longus). It wraps along the lateral aspect of the cuboid bone and inserts at the bottom of the foot. Extensor tendons run in the principal direction of the main muscle and are only utilized for pull.

- *Muscle fasciae* are connective tissue sheaths that envelope individual muscles or muscle groups. This allows multiple muscles to glide past each other without friction.

- *Tendon sheaths* are gliding tunnels that improve the gliding function and guiding of a tendon. The structure of a tendon sheath is similar to that of a joint capsule. The outer layer (stratum fibrosum) consists of connective tissue; the inner layer (stratum synoviale) secretes a type of joint lubricant and improves gliding function.

- *Bursae* (bursae synoviales) have the function of protecting a muscle that wraps directly around a bone.

- *Sesamoid bones* can be found where there is particular pressure on a tendon. They are embedded at the point where the tendon changes direction. There they form a synovial joint together with the underlying bone, to decrease friction. The patella is the largest sesamoid bone.

- The function of sesamoid cartilage is to cover a tendon without embedded bone.

- Between the individual muscles are fatty compounds (corpora adiposa). They also improve the gliding function.

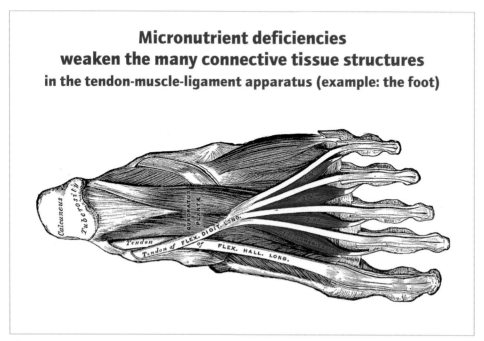

**Micronutrient deficiencies
weaken the many connective tissue structures**
in the tendon-muscle-ligament apparatus (example: the foot)

Fig. 34

3.5   Joints

In order for the body to move, individual bones must be connected to each other and have the ability to telescope. The *joints (articulationes)* are the basis for this movement. They link a large number of the more than 200 skeletal bones.

Joints can be classified according to their degree of mobility. In this regard we differentiate between *uniaxial, biaxial,* and *triaxial* to *multiaxial joints.*

The material found between the bones additionally differentiates different types of joints.

- In the case of fibrous joints (syndemosis) with connective tissue, or cartilaginous joints (synchondrosis) consisting of hyaline cartilage, movement potential is rather limited. The elastic effect is more prevalent here. These joints are also referred to as false joints (synarthrosis). Fibrous joints connect two bones that move against each other with connective tissue. These are uninterrupted joints. They are syndesmosis, gomphosis or suture.

- Cartilaginous joints connect bones that move against each other with cartilage. This can occur as synchondrosis via hyaline cartilage or as symphysis.

- Larger motion sequences can only be executed with true joints (diarthrosis). These are characterized by two bone ends (epyphysis), which together form the joint ball and socket.

- Synovial fluid (synovial) decreases friction between the cartilage-covered joint surfaces. It is contained in a joint capsule (capsula articularis) whose taut tissue holds the joint together.

In addition there are as-needed mechanisms such as ligaments (ligamenta), cushioning disks (disci or menisci articulares), joint margins (labra articularia), etc.

At this point we will exemplify by taking a look at only two joints: the lumbar spine, the knee joint, with the effects of specific micronutrients for structuring and stabilization.

Synovial joints

Synovial joints are also referred to as *free motion joints*. They facilitate a greater range of motion. A joint consists of at least two moveable bodies that are most often covered with hyaline cartilage. Occasionally they are also coveredwith fibro cartilage or connective tissue with elements of fibro cartilage.

This cartilage cover is approximately 2-5 mm thick and allows the two joint moveable bodies -ball and socket- to glide on top of each other or against each other. To make the sequence of this process frictionless, existing gaps between the moveable bodies are filled in with fatty tissue or villi (synovial villi) or folds of the joint capsule's inner membrane (membranan synovialis).

In some places, such as the temporomandibular joint, this also occurs via fibrocartilaginous disks (discus) or, as in the knee joint, with variously shaped menisci.

A remaining capillary gap between the joint *capsule (capsula articularis)* and the joint-forming bone ends is referred to as *cavitas articularis*. So-called *acetabular lips* (labrum articulare) consisting of a fibrocartilaginous rim help to even out the usually smaller joint socket to better surround the ball.

A sometimes taut and sometimes flaccid joint capsule is attached directly to the moveable bodies of the joint adjacent to the cartilage surfaces. It consists of an inner (membrana synovialis) and an outer layer (membrana fibrosa). The inner layer contains nerve fibers and blood vessels and is composed of loose connective tissue. This is also where the previously mentioned villi and folds are located. The outer layer consists of taut connective tissue and is interspersed with a meshwork of nerve fibers. Strong lateral bands often reinforce it. In some places the outer joint capsule is so thin that the inner membrane can bulge out. This is where the synovial fluid that is constantly secreted by the inner membrane is contained. It covers the joint surfaces with a slimy coating, thereby facilitating the gliding of the moveable bodies.

Knee joint

A complex joint – the knee joint – is located between the femur, the tibia and the patella. It is the largest joint in the human body. There is a lot of pressure on the knee, particularly when it is bent. This often causes degenerative changes resulting in pain that can only be relieved with an artificial knee.

The irregular joint surfaces of thigh and tibia are evened out by a relatively thick cartilage cover, as well as two fibrocartilaginous rings, the *menisci*, thereby enlarging the area for force absorption. The patella is also a part of the knee. It is the largest sesamoid bone in the body and is held in place by the patellar ligament.

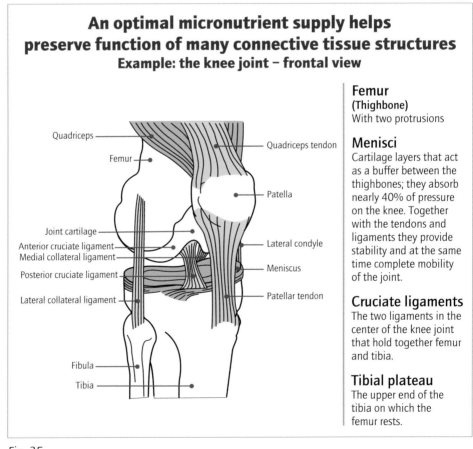

An optimal micronutrient supply helps preserve function of many connective tissue structures
Example: the knee joint – frontal view

Quadriceps
Femur
Quadriceps tendon
Patella
Joint cartilage
Anterior cruciate ligament
Medial collateral ligament
Lateral condyle
Posterior cruciate ligament
Meniscus
Lateral collateral ligament
Patellar tendon
Fibula
Tibia

Femur
(Thighbone)
With two protrusions

Menisci
Cartilage layers that act as a buffer between the thighbones; they absorb nearly 40% of pressure on the knee. Together with the tendons and ligaments they provide stability and at the same time complete mobility of the joint.

Cruciate ligaments
The two ligaments in the center of the knee joint that hold together femur and tibia.

Tibial plateau
The upper end of the tibia on which the femur rests.

Fig. 35

We differentiate between a *femorotibial joint*, where the shin comes into contact with the femur, and a *femoropatellar joint*, where the patella comes into contact with the femur.

The *lateral bands* (ligamenta collaterale tibiale and fibulare) that guide the movements in the knee joint are strong, as well as the *cruciate ligaments* (ligamenta cruciatum anterius and posterius). The latter prevent hyperextension of the knee.

The muscles that move the knee joint include, i.a. for extension, the four-headed thigh muscle (m. quadriceps femoris), for flexion, the two-headed thigh muscle, the semimembranosus muscle, a thigh muscle that stretches from the tuber ischii to the popliteal fossa and to the shin bone, the semitendinosus muscle, a muscle that also stretches from the tuber ischii to the shin bone. While the two-headed thigh musce (m. biceps femoris) rotates the lower leg to the outside (external rotation), the semimembranosus muscle and semitendinosus muscle rotate the lower leg to the inside.

An optimal micronutrient concentration helps maintain joint function
Structure of the knee joint

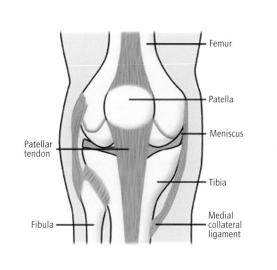

Joint cartilage
The cartilage layer that covers the ends of the bones in all true joints, and provides smooth gliding as well as cushioning.

Joint capsule
It envelops true joints and limits their movement. It helps hold together individual joint structures, thereby stabilizing the joint.

Synovium
A layer of tissue that lines the inside of the joint capsule. It produces the liquid joint fluid (synovia) that eases the gliding motion of joint surfaces.

Femur
Patella
Meniscus
Patellar tendon
Tibia
Fibula
Medial collateral ligament

Fig. 36

In the area of menisci, which consist of connective tissue with collagen fibers and embedded cartilage cells, perpetual overuse or poorly coordinated movement causes injuries. In doing so the crescent-shaped medial meniscus is affected twenty times more often than the circular lateral meniscus. An injury can be either a vertical tear or an avulsion. A meniscus can be surgically removed as long as the capsular rim is intact. A meniscus-like tissue is formed that takes over the function of the meniscus.

Important information

In addition to supporting functional and strong musculature, a sufficient supply of cellular micronutrients can verifiably protect from degeneration.

3.6 Vertebrae

Vertebrae in fact differ in their structure, but most have a common basic two-part structure: the larger cylindrical part is the vertebrae as the actual building block of the column. The vertebral arch connects to the vertebral body and on both sides consists of a pair of pedicles and a lamina, as well as a spinous process, two transverse processes and four articular processes. (A process is an outgrowth or protrusion of bony tissue.)

Weak spot intervertebral discs

The intervertebral discs have two functions: they connect the vertebrae with each other and they buffer impact and pressure caused by movement and lifting weight. Injuries, perpetual weight bearing and age-related wear can damage the intervertebral discs and can cause them to pop out of place (intervertebral disc prolapse). Most of the stress is on the lower back, which is why back pain most often originates with the intervertebral discs of the lumbar spine (low back pain).

Vertebral joints

- *Intervertebral dics:* Between any two vertebrae (1) lies one intervertebral disc (2) consisting of cartilage tissue, whose function it is to absorb shock and pressure caused by movement and weightbearing. The strength of intervertebral discs varies depending on the area of the back. Those between the lumbar vertebrae are thickest.

- *Ligaments:* the discs are connected by fibrous strands that stretch along the entire spinal column: the ligaments (e.g. anterior (3) and posterior (4) longitudinal ligament, interspinous ligament (5). The anterior longitudinal ligament runs on the ventral side (stomach), the anterior on the dorsal side (back).

- *Joint processes:* the two lower (6) and upper (7) joint processes of each vertebra are always connected to the adjacent vertebra.

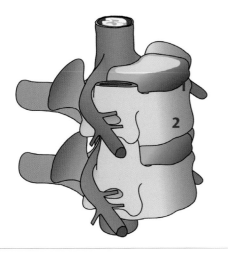

Optimal micronutrient concentrations stabilize connective tissue structures of the vertebrae and intervertebral discs

1 Vertebral body

2 Intervertebral disc

Fig. 37

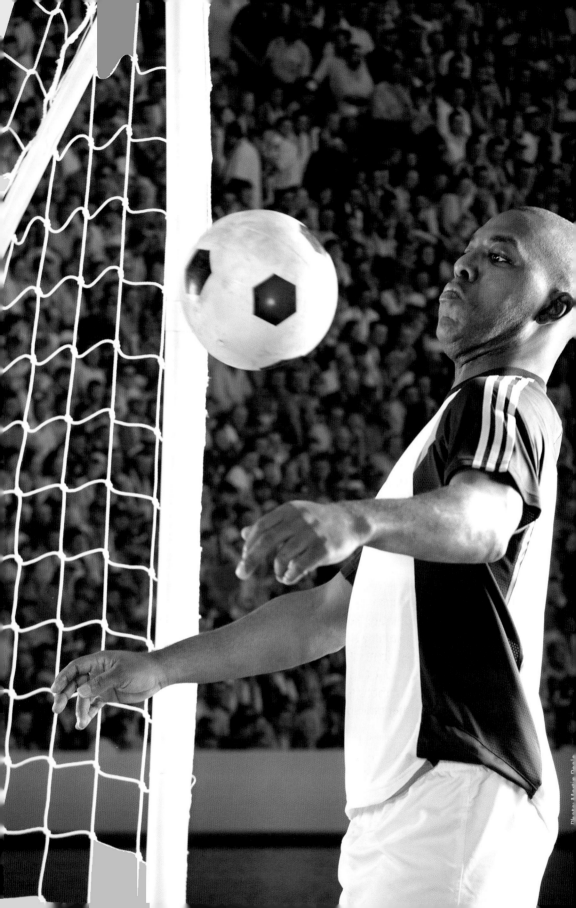

4 The role of micronutrients with respect to body tissue and body functions

4.1 Protection from degenerative diseases (e.g. osteoarthritis and the like)

For athletes the long-term preservation and friction-less functioning of joints in particular is a prerequisite for athletic performance. Recreational and competitive sports can cause damage to the musculoskeletal system. It is common knowledge that intensive athletic activity affects the occurrence of degenerative arthropathy and loss of elasticity in the tendon and ligament apparatus. "No pain, no gain" – at least without high-quality micronutrients.

The up to now by scientists often repudiated link between definite long-term micronutrient deficiencies and increasing injuries, deformation of joints to the point of arthrosis (e.g. shoulder, knee, ankle et al), has so far undergone little scientific testing. Our experience clearly shows that a good cellular micronutrient balance can not only produce the optimal development of physical performance, but also improve the maintenance of bradytrophic tissue structures (tendons, ligaments, cartilage).

Other autologous factors such as familial disposition, stress capacity of cartilage, axial relationships, coordinative abilities, talent, body weight, gender or metabolic disorders,can of course also play a role. Additionally injuries caused by an external force resulting in altered joint stability and mobility must also be taken into consideration. Injury risk varies from sport to sport. Sports with quick directional changes and physical contact (e.g. soccer, team handball, basketball) pose a higher injury risk than other ball sports.

All sports, however, have one thing in common: An optimal supply of micronutrients can verifiably reduce injury risk and lead to a performance increase.

Specific micronutrients for joint health in prevention and therapy for athletes

Intensive training sessions without a specific micronutrient supply inevitably lead to extreme wear on joint cartilagein the long-term. Next to basic amino acids which, based on newer findings, are being used to generate energy (see pg. 82-85) and therefore are no longer sufficiently available for the development of the many connective tissue structures, chondroitin and glucosamine sulfate are essential building blocks of the cartilage metabolism. Both substances can arrest cartilage degeneration. Glucosamine is the main building block for proteoglycan synthesis.

Background information

Proteoglycans arecartilage structures that expand through water absorption and are responsible for the cushioning effect of cartilage. At the same time they also nourish it. All essential amino sugars of proteoglycans, starting with glucosamine, are created in the body.

This is how micronutrients protect the musculoskeletal apparatus

Glucosamine sulfate (GS) and chondroitin sulfate (CS) promote cartilage development and regeneration of the cartilage matrix (anabolic effect).

Synovial activity also improves. The two joint nutrients promote absorption of L-proline (an essential amino acid, see pg. 273) andofsulfurous components into the joints, thereby strengthening collagen fibers. At the same time the activity of cartilage and collagen-building enzymes is diminished. Numerous studies and meta analyses with glucosamine sulfate (dosage: 1500 mg/day) and chondroitin sulfate (800-1200 mg/day) substantiate reduction of pain and swelling and improved joint mobility in gonarthrosis therapy (see Matheson et all, 2003).

S-adenosylmethionine (SAM) is produced in homocysteine metabolism from the essential amino acid L-methionine. Next to several other amino acids, methionine plays a major role in the development of many connective tissue structures (ligaments, tendons) and is indispensible to the development of cartilage. An insufficient supply of methionine can quickly occur during intensive training sessions and is increasingly involved in the energy metabolism. A shortage increases the loss of elasticity in the tendon and ligament apparatus. The targeted supply of a high-quality amino acid blend for the retention of these and other important amino acids is urgently recommended (see pg. 95), particularly with regard to prevention.

Dosage and length of use

In therapy SAM is used as an oral dose of 800-1200 mg/day during initial treatment of knee, hip or spinalinflammation. The pain-reducing and anti-inflammatory effect has been proven in numerous studies of SAM in several double blind multicenter studies.

The following table shows supply recommendations for several micronutrients that support joint mobility through prevention and several mono preparationsthat are takenseparately.

Table 1: Recommended dosage

Micronutrient	Prevention	Therapy
Glucosamine sulfate	1,500 mg (e.g. 2 x 750 mg/day) as interval therapy during high-exertion phases (e.g. competition preparation)	1,500 mg (2 x 750 mg/day) for 2-3 months, then a three-week break from therapy
Chondroitin sulfate	400-1,200 mg (e.g. 2 x 400 mg/day) as interval therapy during high-exertion phases (e.g. competition preparation)	800-1,200 mg (e.g. 3 x 400 mg/day) for 2-3 months, then a three-week break from therapy
S-adenosylmethionine (SAM), degradation product of the amino acid methionine	No supply advisable (only in an adequate concentration of a high-quality amino acid blend)	Orally: 800-1,200 mg SAM, but should be given intravenously in cases of acute inflammatory arthritis.

These specific joint nutrients make particular sense for interval therapy during phases of intensive training over a year. However, it is our experience that these should be adapted to the sport-specific training and competition phases. Ideally newly developed markers for lab diagnostics that can be used for early detection, but also for follow-up and therapy monitoring should be used (see box).

Background information

New lab parameters (pyridinium crosslinks and COMP) offer better clinical diagnostics in the prevention and therapy of musculoskeletal damage. *COMP* (cartilage oligometric matrix protein) is a specific lab parameter for joint cartilage damage with inflammatory and degenerative changes, such as beginning osteoarthritis. The *pyridinoline crosslinks* in urine (see pg. 107-109) are currently considered the best indicators of additional parameters for the assessment of disturbed cartilage and bone metabolism. We had these measured in each of 100 competitive athletes in addition to other immunological and cellular micronutrient concentrations.

4.2   Metabolism

Basic information

The entirety of all biochemical reactions within the organism is referred to as metabolism. Here the nutrients supplied to the body are turned into mechanical activity (muscle) and warmth. A portion is also used for the composition of autologous substances.

Carbohydrates, fats and proteins make up the largest portion of converted substances. Next to that are smaller amounts of trace elements, vitamins and hormones. Trace elements are inorganic bonds or ions that primarily support chemical reactions as so called *coenzymes*. *Vitamins* are organic substances that cannot be manufactured by humans or animals, but must be ready for consumption. *Hormones* by contrast are messengers that only exist in multi-cellular life forms.

Within the metabolism we differentiate between anabolic and catabolic metabolism.

- In the anabolic phase nutrients are continuously converted to organic substances or substances whose combustion creates energy.

- In the catabolic phase these substances are released through diuresis, perspiration or exhalation of carbon dioxide.

While the anabolic phase is dominant during adolescence, the phases are balanced during adulthood. Constructive and energy metabolisms involve very different processes. They use energyas a rule. Constructive metabolism includes all reactions that end with a new cell element, such as lipids in biomembranes or actin in cytoskeleton. While constructive metabolism in the narrower sense refers only to the synthesis of building blocks for cell growth, energy metabolism produces all of the "replacement building blocks", thus taking care of the repair and replacement of defective or used up elements. Additionally it provides energy for all metabolic processes.

Metabolic processes take place in different steps under the influence of enzymes. These are biological catalysts that control, or rather speed upchemical processes by, on the one hand, lowering the temperature required for a reaction, but also not changing themselves.

A balanced metabolism provides the human body with a state of equilibrium of physiological functions, stable blood pressure, body temperature and chemical composition within the internal fluid. Maintaining body function requires a minimal amount of energy referred to as *basic metabolic rate*.

Optimizing the metabolism – activation of enzymes through micronutrients

Enzymes cause all of the metabolic reactions taking place in our body. Biochemical processes would not take place without enzymes, the so-called *metabolic catalysts*. However, most enzymes can only accomplish their metabolic work with a sufficient supply of micronutrients of vitamins and minerals. The blatant cellular micronutrient deficiencies vastly limit the metabolic activity in such a way that these athletes exhibit a much higher predisposition to infection and injury (see pg. 126-129).

An insufficient supply of micronutrients keeps the entire energy production process from functioning optimally. The athletes' regeneration ability decreases and predisposition to injury, specifically with respect to various minor injuries, clearly increases so that training continuity is hardly a given and a competitive athlete is no longer able to meet his potential.

Background information

The optimization of the metabolism requires accurate diagnosis. Each individual micronutrient has highly specialized functions within our metabolism (see pg. 246-277). For the purpose of assessing micronutrient requirements and the appropriate dosage for optimal metabolic function it is, next to several blood parameters, the micronutrient concentration in erythrocytes that is particularly well suited. Routine blood serum analyses do not provide any exact information (see pg. 34-39). Combinations of individual micronutrient formulations are the result of a detailed nutrition analysis, intracellular blood test, additional protocol sheets and a database with results of competitive and recreational athletes.

There are few institutions in Europe that regularly conduct intracellular micronutrient measurements. However, the evaluation and interpretation of the respective micronutrient analyses for competitive athletes is much more important due to an adequate existing database.

The principle of super compensation

The principle of the optimal training load-recovery relation is one of the most important training principles. Each training session leads to a catabolic reaction of the metabolism. The organism rapidly uses essential resources (various protein structures, etc.) to withstand the physical exertion.

After a while it rebuilds the substances beyond the old base level. The rebuilding phase is called an anabolic reaction of the metabolism. This state of increased energetic capacity is referred to as *super compensation*. It is a model that is the subject of much controversy in sports science circles. The training affects a number of the body's regulatory systems:

- the central nervous system,

- the autonomic nervous system,

- the neuromuscular system,

- the energy processes,

- the cardio respiratory system,

- the detoxification system and

- the hormone system

The regeneration period of these individual systems and processes varies. It depends largely on the energy producing processes. If there is evidence of important fundamental micronutrient deficiencies, autologous structural proteins are rapidly incorporated into the metabolism, which are then no longer available for the maintenance of various vital connective tissue functions (ligaments, tendons, cartilage). Competitive athletes with substantial micronutrient supply deficiencies demonstrate a considerably higher injury risk (see pg. 101, 102, 108).

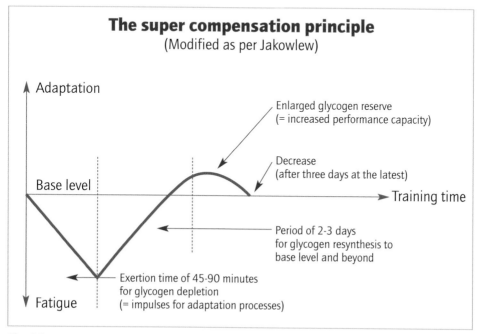

Fig. 38

Autologous resources are exhausted

The competitive athlete can utilize autologous structural proteins for energy purposes for a limited period of time. But for the long-term this means that additional increases in micronutrient deficiencies will cause a significant restriction of the entire energy system, so that after a period of time (this can occur weeks or months later) the athlete will complain of various ailments. It is exactly here that the significance of customized micronutrient formulations becomes apparent. Based on the blood test results from the COMP method (cartilage, oligometric matrix protein) and the results from the pyridinium cross links, results from competitive athletes show initial interesting correlations between degenerative changes in various connective tissues and micronutrient deficiencies.

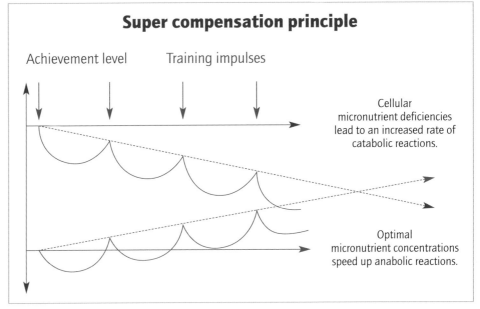

Fig. 39

An insufficient cellular micronutrient concentration affects the principle of super compensation in a variety of ways. In competitive athletes with blatant micronutrient deficiencies excessive intensive training can cause different enzymatic shortages in the area of energy supply and thus long-term performance decreases.

4.3 Revolutionary findings on the energy supply and micronutrient balance in athletes

The more intensive or extensive the physical activity in recreational or competitive sports the higher the need for energy-providing macronutrients (e.g. carbohydrates) and also for catalysts of our metabolism, the minerals, trace elements and vitamins. Micronutrients play an important role in many catabolic and anabolic metabolic processes (e.g. building muscle, storing muscle glycogen). In addition they are also involved in the regulation of muscle contractions, transmission of nerve impulses, coordination, and acid-base balance. Energy and micronutrient requirements increase significantly during athletic training.

Even a minor under-supply of micronutrients can have an adverse effect on physical and psychological performance. Significant cellular micronutrient deficiencies were found by athletes with a balanced diet, that lead to a variety of ailments. In terms of optimal metabolic function and physical fitness, athletes are more dependent on this than non-athletes.

Brief characterization of the energy metabolism

The energy required for the listed functions in cells is won through gradual oxidation of the following nutrients:

- Sugar, e.g. grape sugar (glucose),

- Fats (particularly fatty acids) and

- Proteins (amino acids).

Newer research shows that proteins are increasingly drawn on for energy production during intensive and extensive training sessions. The danger here is long-term loss of important structural protein substances resulting in their limited availability to develop various connective tissue structures (tendons, ligaments, cartilage) and support the immune system.

Biological oxidations can be compared to combustion processes, however they occur without flames and at relatively low temperatures. *Oxidation* is a general term for the loss of electrons (é). In the process high-energy nutrients turn into low-energy bonds like urea, CO_2 and H_2O.

Principals of energy supply in the skeletal muscles during physical activity

During physical exertion in sports energy requirements increase due to the energy needed for muscle contractions. Depending on the type and the intensity of the sport, this metabolic increase can be significantly higher than the resting metabolic rate. Thus the energy requirements of an athlete sprinting at maximum speed show a thousand-fold maximum increase per time unit. Also, during a short distance sprint the increased metabolic rate begins suddenly andends after only 10-20 sec.

Here, too, the principal is put into practice that energy that is released incrementally during oxidation of nutrients does not go directly to the cell processes requiring energy, but is first stored in high-energy phosphate bonds. The two most important high-energy phosphate bonds are:

- **ATP** (adenosine triphosphate) and

- **KP** (creatine phosphate)

The entire amount of energy from both high-energy bonds is enough for approximately 20 maximum muscle contractions (approx. 6-10 sec.). But since maximum physical performance requires significantly more muscle contractions, chemical reactions must take place within the active muscle cell that will supply energy to refill the ATP and KP energy stores. The subsequent energy supply occurs through the biological oxidation of nutrients. There are basically two ways for the biological oxidation to take place:

- **Aerobic oxidation** of nutrients with the use of oxygen, and

- **Anaerobic oxidation** of carbohydrates (mainly glucose) without oxygen.

Aerobic oxidation

Aerobic oxidation takes place in the mitochondria ("cell power house"). For this purpose oxygen and pyruvate (pyruvic acid) must be transported to the mitochondria. Conversely the ATP that was produced as well as the CO_2 and H_2O that formed leave the mitochondria.

The *mitochondria* are the cell's energy delivery service and are therefore also called the *powerhouses*. Nutrients such as sugar and fat that reach the cell are burned in the mitochondria with the aid of oxygen. Similar to the nucleus, mitochondria are also enclosed in a double-layer membrane (see Fig. 40). The intermediate fluid is comparable to the extracellular fluid located between the individual cells. Their inner membrane is heavily folded, thus providing a large surface area. The mitochondria themselves are long filaments that move in a circular or winding motion. They occur in various numbers in all cells with the exception of red blood cells (erythrocytes).

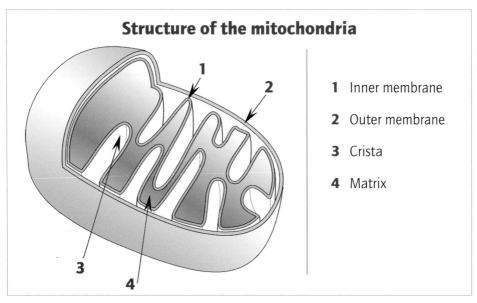

Structure of the mitochondria

1 Inner membrane

2 Outer membrane

3 Crista

4 Matrix

Fig. 40

Aerobic oxidation occurs in enzyme-controlled levels, which in turn consist of multi-step reactions. With respect to grape sugar storage – glycogen –, located in the muscle cell, there are five different catabolic steps:

1. The *glycogenolysis*: Here the respective glycogen molecule at the end is split off from the chain-like glycogen molecule consisting of glycogen molecules.

2. The *glycolysis* (breakdown of glucose): Incremental breakdown of glucose into pyruvic acid with the aid of numerous enzymes (pyruvate).

3. Formation of *activated acetic acid* (aectyl-CoA): In order for pyruvate to be used for further aerobic breakdown it must first be converted to acetic acid with the use of several enzymes and coenzymes. This formation of activated acetic acid represents a key reaction in the oxidative breakdown of nutrients. Not only glucose but also fatty acids and amino acids (protein building blocks) are processed aerobically during energy gain via acetyl-CoA.

4. *Citrate cycle*: The activated acetic acid is broken down in the citric acid cycle.

5. The respiratory chain consists of an electron transfer protein sequence. The respiratory chain is also referred to as the *electron transfer chain*.

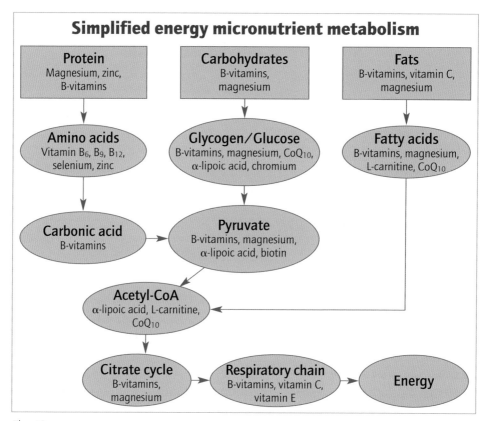

Fig. 41

Depending on energy demand, the enzyme-controlled steps during aerobic energy supply (activation of acetic acid, citrate cycle and respiratory chain) are partially sped up or slowed down through complex reactions. Summing up, aerobic oxidation is ultimately characterized by the fact that the hydrogen in nutrients (and its electrons) is transferred to the oxygen and during this reaction sequence the de-energized bonds water and CO_2 form. In the process nearly 100% of the energy contained in the glycogen molecule is released and under standard conditions approximately 40% of it can be stored in high-energy phosphate ATP.

Conclusion: Micronutrient deficiencies in the energy supply of carbohydrate and fat metabolism can lead to an enzyme blockage. The energy supply then comes from autologous amino acids that are subsequently no longer sufficiently available for the important connective tissue structures (ligaments, tendons, cartilage).

Anaerobic oxidation

The much larger share of the energy required during physical activity, particularly during extended periods of exertion, is supplied via aerobic oxidation of nutrients. The second way to supply energy – *the anaerobic oxidation* – is tapped into when current energy requirements cannot be met by aerobic oxidation. During anaerobic oxidation energy is supplied from glucose that is broken down via the already mentioned glycolysis method. Up to the formation of acetic acid the reaction steps for anaerobic and aerobic oxidation are the same. If the glycolysis (glucose scission) is boosted due to a strong increase in energy demand, more acetic acid (pyruvate) accumulates than can be processed oxidatetively, and *lactate* (lactic acid) forms. However, the developing energy amounts are very limited and only briefly available. High lactate formation inevitably leads to muscle fatigue and the organism is forced to reduce activity or stop altogether.

Enzymes of anaerobic oxidation (glycolysis) are localized in the cell plasma (sarcoplasm). Therefore the supply of anaerobic energy takes place in the immediate vicinity of the myofibril in the muscle cell. It was previously thought that only 15% of the accumulating lactate would be resynthesized to glucose in the liver during energy use. But many scientists from various scientific fields challenge this vehemently. They are of the opinion that this portion is considerably larger and can also result from amino acids. This regeneration of glucose is called *gluconeogenesis*.

While the energy from high-energy phosphates is only enough for a maximal exertion time of 6 seconds, during the supply of anaerobic lactate energy this time period is approximately 60 seconds, and during the supply of aerobic energy from glycogen it increases to 60 minutes. Fatty acids as aerobic energy suppliers increase the maximum exertion time to significantly more then 60 minutes. Insufficient replenishment of the glycogen stores in liver and musculature after intensive stress due to substantial micronutrient deficiencies very quickly leads to short-term activation of autologous amino acids that are then no longer sufficiently available for connective tissue synthesis of ligaments, tendons and cartilage.

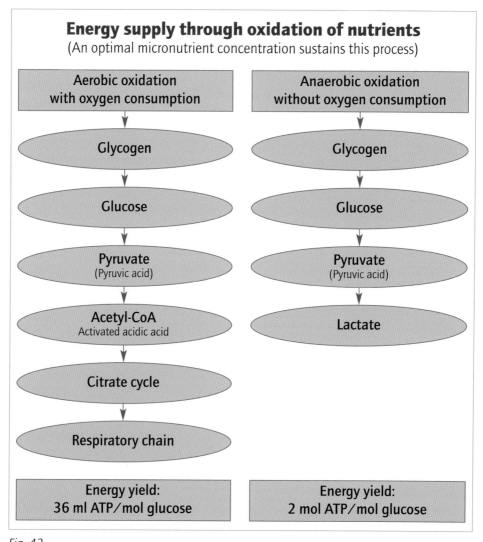

Fig. 42

Increasing micronutrient deficiencies paralyze metabolic energy production

The cellular blood tests of endurance athletes (soccer, team handball, triathletes, marathon runners, et al, see pg. 24, 28-31) show considerable micronutrient deficiencies. This shows that certain metabolic energy supply processes are progressing slower or inadequately. These prevent, among other things, the optimal development of endurance capacity due to various physiological processes and delay the regeneration ability after intensive exertion. The athlete is unable to adequately refill his glycogen stores in the liver and musculature so that subsequent energy-supplying processes occur from protein structures that are then no longer sufficiently available for the basic synthesis of the various connective tissue structures (see pg. 86, 95).

We are only examining athletes here that verifiably already have a balanced diet according to German Nutrition Society criteria. The cellular deficiencies with a diet that is not balanced are by far greater, and this is usually the case with recreational athletes. Our experiences during the past few years, particularly from our last clinical study with 100 athletic women who already had a very balanced diet, show significant micronutrient deficiencies after four months of training three times a week for 40 minutes. In competitive athletes these increasing deficiencies seriously restrict the entire energy and anabolic metabolism. The consequences are increased loss of elasticity in the tendon-ligament apparatus and long-tem degeneration of cartilage structures. Initial preliminary testing of competitive athletes with MRT-imaging has already shown the start of a trend in individual cases. However, long-term testing over the course of several years is necessary.

The importance of high-quality amino acids for the energy metabolism

Our special blood tests from recent years show blatant deficiencies of high-quality amino acids, even though these athletes had a good nutrition analyses according to German Nutrition Society criteria.

Higher requirements during intensive and/or extensive training sessions have increasingly resulted in basic amino acids (i.a. arginine, methonine, glycine, proline, etc.) being tapped into for energy supply. They are then no longer sufficiently available for the various connective tissue functions. The amino acid

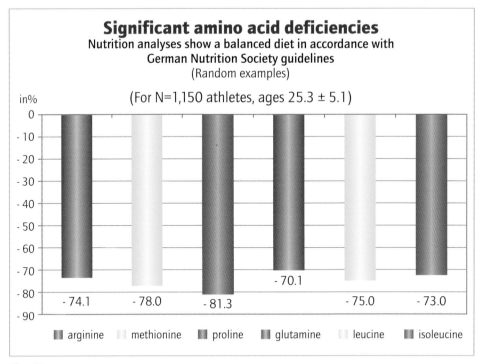

Fig. 43

metabolism diagram shows how autologous protein structures can be drawn on via resynthesis during the citrate cycle during intensive training sessions. Recent

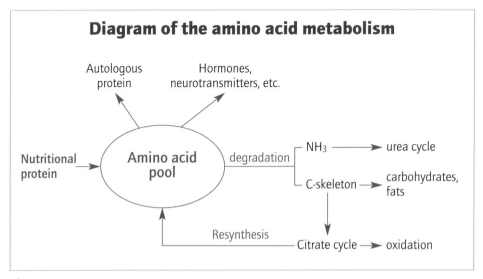

Fig. 44

tests also show the increasing significance of high-quality amino acids for the energy metabolism during intensive training and competition phases.

Next to a long-term degeneration of bradytrophic connective tissue structures (decreased elasticity of the ligament-tendon apparatus and cartilage synthesis) this process can also lead to susceptibility to infection and fluctuating performance (also see super compensation model, pg 78).

Creatine phosphate stores are very important for "explosiveness" (e.g. during maximal sprint exertion for up to 6 sec.), especially in ball sports like team handball and soccer with lots of quick directional changes, but also in other sports. Here, too, a specific supply of high-quality amino acids (AM formula blend) can speed up the refilling of KP stores.

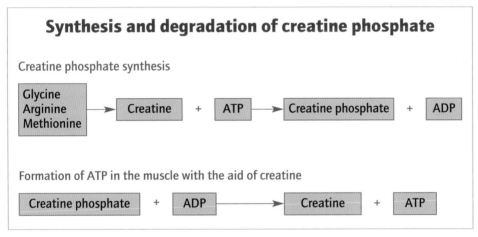

Fig. 45

Increasing deficits of micronutrients paralyze the energy system concerning the metabolism

Based on our longtime experience, an optimal athletic diet is far from sufficient for all of these complex energy systems.

Even the up to now frequently offered recommendations by scientists in the area of micronutrient dosage are no longer up to date.

Initial research with the aid of newly developed methods (pyridinium crosslinks and COMP) and initial measurements taken from competitive athletes show a link between the long-term degeneration of bradytrophic connective tissue structures (ligaments, tendons, cartilage) and the micronutrient concentration.

Autologous amino acids are increasingly drawn upon for energy production during intensive and extensive training sessions and thus are no longer sufficiently available for synthesis and stabilization in the tendon-ligament apparatus. Cellular micronutrient deficiencies can also create an energy supply shortfall, again resulting in the use of autologous structural proteins for the metabolism.

4.4   Amino acids – life's building blocks

An optimal supply of amino acids guarantees performance and protection from injuries. Proteins are basic building blocks of all the body's cells and control all biochemical processes in the body. As basic building blocks of muscle fiber and as scleroprotein and protective protein of cartilage matrix, bones, tendons and dermis, proteins are the most important structural elements in the body.

A constant synthesis and breakdown of proteins takes place inside the organism. Amino acids are basic building blocks of proteins. We have only a limited amino acid store of approximately 120 grams that is located in the blood plasma and mostly in the musculature and in cellular structures. Since the organism is not capable of storing sufficient amounts of amino acids, a daily high-quality protein supply through nutrition is in order.

Essential and nonessential amino acids

The human body is not able to produce eight of a total of 22 amino acids on its own. These essential amino acids must be supplied through nutrition. In the meantime a few semi-essential amino acids have been identified, a regular supply of which is necessary to carry out important functions in our metabolism.

To what extent the traditional classification of *essential* and *nonessential* amino acids will be maintained is however debatable since some research has shown that the boundaries between these two groups are sometimes fluid. We have been able to show that even nonessential amino acids can be essential in certain situations.

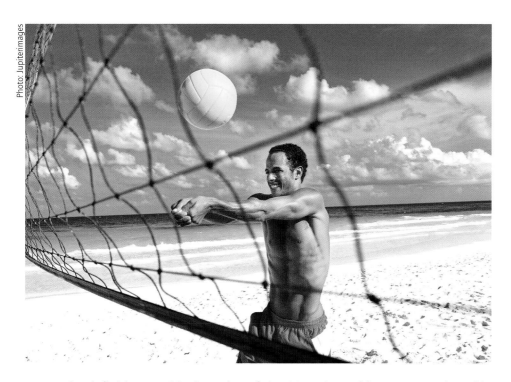

As per the definition, at this time nine of the 20 amino acids are non-replaceable (essential):

- Essential amino acids include: histidine, valine, leucine, isoleucine, lysine, methionine, phenylalanine, threonine, tryptophan.

- Conditionally essential amino acids include: arginine, glycine, cysteine, glutamine, tyrosine, serine, taurine.

- Nonessential, yet still important amino acids are: alanine, aspartic acid, asparagine, glutamine acid, ornithine, proline.

Tasks and functions of some amino acids

Amino acids in natural proteins always exist in L-shapes. The L designates the molecule's spatial structure. With few exceptions, only L-amino acids from the body can be used. When we speak of amino acids here, we always refer to the L-amino acids (e.g. glutamine = L-glutamine). Further details about the various tasks and functions of amino acids can be found in the appendix, pg. 264ff.

Table 2: Tasks and functions of various amino acids

Arginine	Energy metabolism, stimulation of immune system, creatine synthesis, release of growth hormones, ammonia detoxification (urea cycle), supports regeneration ability.
Methionine (sulphurous AS)	As a precursor to SAM (S-adenosylmethionine) it is indispensible to the formation of cartilage, L-gluthathione; an important protein building block.
Glutamine	Building of muscle, energy production, important nutrient for the intestinal mucosa, improves memory, stabilizes blood sugar level and immune system.
Glutamic acid	Improves concentration and performance, memory.
Leucine, isoleucine, valine (BCAA)	Energy production, ammonia detoxification, protection from premature fatigue in sports, builds muscle.
Lysine	Carnitinesynthesis, stimulates immune system.
Asparagine/aspartic acid	Energy production, builds up immune system.
Glycine	Stimulates immune system, formation of immunoglobulin, detoxifying function of the liver.
Histidine	Production of red blood cells.
Taurine	Strengthens immune system, protects tissue from oxidative damage caused by free radicals.
Cysteine (NAC)	Protects cells from free radicals, strengthens immune system.
Cystine	Supports formation of skin and hair.
Alanine	Regulates blood sugar, optimizes muscle energy supply (esp. during endurance workouts).

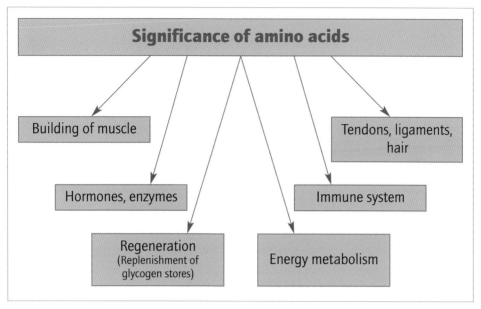

Fig. 46

High-quality amino acids carry out important tasks within the organism, i.a.:

*   During energy metabolism: Synthesis of creatine phosphate; building up glycogen stores; supports combustion of fatty acids;

*   Improved mental and muscular regeneration;

*   Optimal protection from injuries and immune stabilization and

*   Optimal building of bradytrophic tissue structures.

Triumvirate of the BCAA's

The so-called BCAA's, *leucine, isoleucine* and *valine* are indispensable for the building of muscle mass. Especially in sports, BCAA's contribute to energy production. A deficiency of these three amino acids boosts the absorption of tryptophan in the brain, causing the affected individual to tire more quickly.

During intense endurance exertion BCAA's are transformed into glucose, thereby stabilizing the athlete's energy and sugar balance. They improve energy production in endurance sports, decrease lactate build up, delay mental fatigue, promote release of human growth hormone, support the building of muscle and combat the breaking down of muscle mass during long-lasting exertion.

L-arginine and ornithine

With a balanced nutrition approximately 3-6 grams of l-arginine is ingested with food each day. L-arginine is abundant in nuts, seeds, legumes and red meat. Arginine is an alkaline amino acid and with four nitrogen atoms is the most nitric amino acid. L-arginine forms from citrulline during the urea cycle (ammonia synthesis), particularly in the kidneys, but also in other organs and blood cells. L-ornithine is a product of the urea cycle because it originates from arginine during the urea split-off. Tasks and functions of arginine and ornithine are for example:

• increases immune capacity (improved lymphocyte and natural killer cell activity),

• collagen synthesis/wound healing,

• improved regeneration after intensive exertion, as well as

• creatine synthesis (creatine phosphate = energy storing method)

A balanced arginine concentration of an additional up to 5 grams per day can protect from cardiovascular diseases (ADMA – a new cardio vascular risk factor). Arginine should always be supplied in an optimal ratio to the other amino acids.

Conserving autologous reserves

Newer research shows that amino acid use for autologous carbohydrate production (gluconeogenesis) is considerably higher than previously thought. Conservation of the amino acid quota can be achieved by:

• good basic endurance and consequently an efficient fat metabolism,

• carbohydrate intake (40-60 grams per hour of exertion) and

• an amino acid supply (10-15 grams per hour of exertion).

If the athlete has good basic endurance and has a sufficient carbohydrate intake during exertion he is better able to conserve amino acids. However, if the supply of amino acids and carbohydrates is lacking during intensive or longer training sessions, amino acid stores in the muscles and blood drop sharply. Amino acids then are no longer sufficiently available for the formation of muscle, tendons and ligaments as well as the immune system, thereby verifiably increasing injury risk significantly.

Ammonia-lowering amino acids improve regeneration ability

Ammonia is a fatigue factor during short intensive as well as long enduring exertions, which then leads to fatigue especially in muscles and brain.

Recent research shows that elevated ammonia levels during intensive exertion can be brought down more quickly with a supply of amino acids such as aspartic acid, glutamine acid and arginine.

At the same time a good supply of high-quality amino aids, preferably with a high percentage of branched chain amino acids (valine, leucine, isoleucine) and ammonia-lowering amino acids (aspartic acid, arginina, glutamine acid and glutamine) stabilize performance and verifiably reduce injury susceptibility. Optimal, based on its composition, is AM-formula blend.

Amino acids protect connective tissue during major exertion

Since every organ is surrounded by connective tissue a healthy connective tissue is the optimal prerequisite for the efficient, productive performanceof organs. The combined connective tissue of an adult weighs approximately 30 lbs. and connects all of the organs as well as the nerves with each other. Connective tissue structures also connect muscles and bones.

Yet, who isn't familiar with this problem: the many performance-oriented recreational athletes experience increasing problems with the Achilles tendon, the hips, knees, etc. These could be the first signs of weak connective tissue structures that are susceptible during major exertion. Connective tissue structures that are particularly at risk are:

- joint cartilage,

- ligaments and tendons,

- joint capsules and

- intervertebral discs.

Initial onset of problems does not have to occur. Connective tissue can be significantly strengthened with a balanced diet and a targeted supply of amino acids.

Our research with performance-oriented recreational athletes as well as professional athletes showed that specifically these types of ailments are indicative of basic deficiencies of bradytrophic tissue-building amino acids (proline, glycine, lysine, aginine, methionine and cysteine). Many minor problems can be avoided from the start with targeted nutritional restructuring towards foods containing silica and the necessary supplementary use of a high-quality amino acid blend (AM-formula blend).

Letting connective tissue gradually adapt to exertion

Tendons and ligaments connect muscle and bone and are therefore heavily used during every movement. Cartilage structures also protect the bone from direct attrition in the joint area. The strong bradytrophic connective tissue structures so important to an athlete's health and performance require long-term training development. The adjustment time for the various connective tissue structures, especially the tendon-ligament apparatus, to the training load is longer than the adjustment of the cardio vascular system. This should be taken into consideration when planning training.

Apart from long-term training development it is also possible to support connective tissue through sensible nutrition. All the more important are nutritional physiological measures for the specific support of highly stressed connective tissue structures. Connective tissue structures consist of protein (collagen fibers)

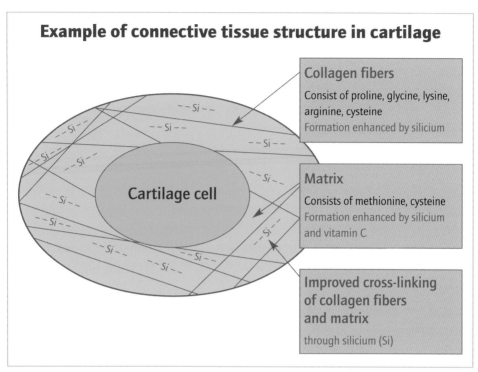

Example of connective tissue structure in cartilage

Cartilage cell

Collagen fibers
Consist of proline, glycine, lysine, arginine, cysteine
Formation enhanced by silicium

Matrix
Consists of methionine, cysteine
Formation enhanced by silicium and vitamin C

Improved cross-linking of collagen fibers and matrix
through silicium (Si)

Fig. 47: Example of bradytrophic connective tissue structure in cartilage

and a matrix of the sulfurous amino acids methionine and cysteine. Cellular micronutrient deficiencies (vitamins, minerals, trace elements) and deficits by amino acids can lead to a weakening of various connective tissue structures. The importance of connective tissue-building amino acids is shown in the illustration Fig 47.

Strong bradytrophic connective tissue structures need silica.

The most important nutrients for strong connective tissue, and thus for strong tendons and ligaments, are amino acids and a diet that is high in silica (e.g. whole grain products, common horsetail extracts, etc.). The central ingredient in silica is *silicium*. Silicium promotes autologous production of fibers and matrix. In addition silicium facilitates an improved crosslink.

For athletes an additional supply is essential.

In view of the variety of biological functions it is obvious that the metabolism must have a constant sufficient supply of the full spectrum of amino acids. This can only be accomplished with a regular re-supply of amino acids from nutritional protein since autologous amino acids are constantly used, or rather broken down into ammonia and subsequently converted to urea in the liver and then expelled as such via the kidneys. It is our experience that autologous protein structures in performance-oriented and top athletes are used energetically in spite of optimal nutrition and thus are no longer available for the regeneration and stability of bradytrophic tissue.

Preliminary test results

Our preliminary tests on 1,150 professional athletes and recreation-oriented competitive athletes showed significant deficiencies in the area of amino acids and cellular micronutrients in spite of a balanced diet. After a detailed nutrition analysis the athletes were given practical recommendations to balance the measured amino acid deficiencies.

In spite of an improved diet subsequent tests did not show an adequate replenishment of important amino acids. The higher the training volume, the greater were the deficiencies in the area of high-quality amino acids and other micronutrients (this is not limited to the so-called *essential* amino acids) with a significant increase in injury risk. The athletes reported an increase in muscular and tendon-ligament problems during the preparatory phase and at the start of the season.

The performance-oriented recreational athletes and the competitive athletes (N = 559) then started taking a specific supply of the AM-formula blend during intensive training phases (20 grams to 3-4 x 20 g, depending on the blood test results) after training sessions and in the evening with dinner. An optimal effect was seen only in the combination with acustomized micronutrient formulation based on our cellular blood test (see pg. 101, 102). Based on our experience, doses of the high-quality protein blend (AM-formula blend) of less than 30 g verifiably do not show a significant effect.

The athletes reported considerably improved reaction ability after training exertion. The various test results of the athletes' immune system showed high stability compared to the group of athletes that had not taken high-quality amino acids and micronutrients. Problems reported by these athletes with respect to the tendon-ligament apparatus were clearly fewer.

The biological valence of protein

The biological valence of a protein results from its amino acid pattern and indicates how much autologous protein is formed from 100 g of nutritional protein. The higher the essential (vital) amino acid content in a protein the more nutritional protein can be converted to autologous protein. A whole egg, as reference value, meets the daily requirements of an adult with 0.5 g per 1000 g of body weight. Its biological valence is 100.

The biologically highest-quality protein from only one protein source, with a valence of 104, is whey protein. Nutritional proteins can be supplemented in their amino acid pattern with a combination of plant and animal protein sources to form a high-quality protein. The highest biological valence of 136 consists of a mix of whole eggand potato (see pg. 213-238, nutritional tips).

Explicit reference should be made here to the importance of the composition of amino acids. Simply providing a high-quality amino acid does not make sense, but rather the composition and ratio of the individual amino acids in a blend is what matters.

Protein powder/whey protein/milk protein/soy protein – which is most effective?

Taking 30-80 g of high-quality amino acids during intensive training and competition phases can give support particularly to the stability of connective tissue structures. Our regular nutrition analyses and cellular blood tests of amino acids show that in spite of a balanced diet professional team handball and soccer players (see pg. 100-102) exhibited considerable deficiencies that led, among other things, to repeated tendon and ligament problems in these players.

A specificsupply is recommended depending on the blood status of the amino acids and the intended training effort. The optimal dosage of a specific supply of basic vitamins, trace elements and minerals also allows for effective absorption.

It is the correct ratio of amino acids to each other that is critical to the usefulness of an amino acid product, rather than the quantity of a few popular amino acids or the overall quantity.

Protein powder

Tasteless amino acids as protein hydrolyzate in powder form are an ideal supplement. We have had positive practical experience with the combined amino acids in the AM-formula blend and many athletes (marathon, triathlon, biathlon, soccer, tennis, team handball) are using it at this time.

The AM-formula blend is an enzymatic hydrolyzate from animal protein with short-chain peptides and L-amino acids of highest purity and quality. It is an almost white, dry, free-flowing powder with nearly neutral smell and taste.

Optimal intake mode: 10-20 g before and 20-30 g after training, respectively, dissolved in sports drinks.

Whey proteins

Next to their high biological valence of 104, whey proteins exhibit better absorption, solubility and gastrointestinal tolerability than comparable, slowly absorbed milk proteins. They possess a particularly high valine, leucine and isoleucine content that can be indirectly metabolized in the energy metabolism.

The so-called PDCAAS (protein digestibility corrected amino acid score) is 100 % for whey protein, an absolute top score. The extremely good absorption causes a quick and high uptake of amino acids in the blood that can then be directly used for the synthesis of muscle protein. If whey protein is further converted to whey isolate it is considered the highest-quality protein from whey. Gentle processing preserves protein components that support the immune system (immunoglobulin). High calcium content is typical. 100 g of whey contain less than 1 g of protein, but it is of particularly high quality.

Milk protein

Compared to the AM-formula blend and whey protein, milk protein (casein) is absorbed very slowly. Milk protein molecules (peptides) are large and must first be broken down into smaller units. It provides long-term support for the building of muscle and contains a high level of glutamine.

Milk protein isolate (ratio casein: lactalbumin = 80 : 20) by comparison is a quickly accessible and slow protein component characterized by a high percentage of branched amino acids (leucine, isoleucine, valine) and glutamine. It contains more than 90% protein, promotes regeneration and is high in calcium.

Soy protein

Soy protein is a protein that is low in branched amino acid content and high in glutamine and isoflavones.

Table 3: Composition of the AM-formula blend

Amino acid	Specifications in g per 100 g protein powder (AM-formula blend)
L-alanine	8.7
L-arginine	8.1
L-aspartic acid	6.0
L-glutamic acid	11.1
L-glycine	20.6
L-histidine	0.6
L-hydroxyproline	1.0
L-isoleucine	11.4
L-leucine	1.6
L-lysine	3.3
L-methionine	3.9
L-phenylalanine	2.1
L-proline	13.3
L-serine	3.1
L-threonine	1.8
L-thyrosine	0.3
L-valine	2.4

The AM-formula blend composition

The composition and combination of amino acids in the AM-formula blend is shown in this table. Numerous tests done with athletes have shown a high level of effectiveness of the amino acids supplied with the AM-formula blend.

Please note: an optimal supplement to the AM-formula blend is the supply of 0.5-11 g of pure whey for stabilization of various connective tissue structures.

4.5 Pilot project – Correlation between a sufficient amino acid concentration, cellular micronutrient balance and injury risk

The correlation between a sufficient supply of high-quality amino acids, an optimal cellular micronutrient concentration and injury rate, particularly during training and competitive exertion without external force, can be seen in the following illustrations. The accompanying research was done with athletes without a specific supply of micronutrients (N = 591) as well as competitive athletes with a targeted supply (N = 559) for a total of three years.

Project execution

The 591 male athlete test subjects, who did not receive a customized micronutrient formulation, consumed an average 3,395 ± 626 cal. The athletes' dosages were in accordance with the German Nutrition Society (see pg. 246-263). The competitive athletes' nutrition analyses corresponded up to 90% with the amounts recommended by the German Nutrition Society for the respective athletic activity. The total energy supply consisted of 58% carbohydrates, 28% fat and 14% protein, whichapproximates recommendations. The average fluid supply was 4.1 ± 1.3 liters. For most micronutrients supply and routine serum blood tests were in a normal range, while cellular analyses (of erythrocytes) of micronutrients (Mg, Zn, Se, B_1, B_2, B_6, B_9) showed definite deficiencies.

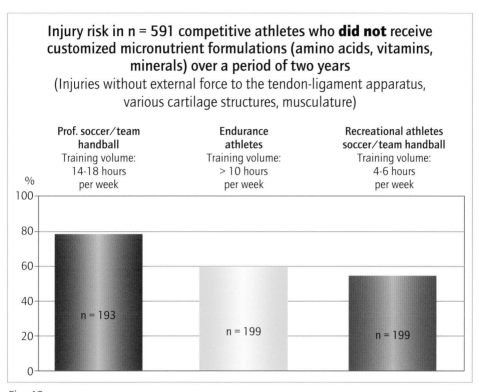

Fig. 48

Table 4: Anthropometric data from a total of 591 competitive athletes who did not receive regular customized micronutrient formulations.

	Age (years)	Height (cm)	Weight (kg)	BMI kg/m²
Total (N = 591)	28.3 ± 8.3	185 ± 4.85	74.8 ± 4.4	21.9

The 559 male athlete test subjects, who did receive individual micronutrient formulations, consumed an average 3,495 ± 526 cal. The competitive athletes' nutrition analyses corresponded up to 90% with the amounts recommended by the German Nutrition Society for the respective athletic activity. The total energy supply consisted of 56% carbohydrates, 29% fat, 15% protein, which approximates recommendations. The average fluid supply was 4.4 ± 1.5 liters. For most micronutrients supply and routine serum blood tests were in a normal range, while cellular analyses (of erythrocytes) of micronutrients (Mg, Zn, Se, B_1, B_2, B_6, B_9) showed definite deficiencies.

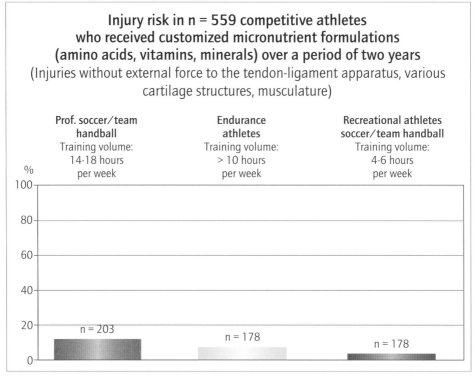

Fig. 49

Table 5: Anthropometric data from a total of 559 competitive athletes who did receive regular customized micronutrient formulations.

	Age (years)	Height (cm)	Weight (kg)	BMI kg/m²
Total (N = 559)	28.1 ± 7.2	184 ± 4.0	75.2 ± 3.9	22.9

Amino acid deficiencies

Blatant deficiencies in amino acids that are important to bradytrophic tissue structures clearly result in an increased injury risk without external force in the athletes we tested. Even the strictly endurance athletes (marathon, triathlon) often complained of various tendon and ligament problems. Blood tests clearly showed a definite deficiency, especially in amino acids that are responsible for the structure and stability of bradytrophic tissue structures. These are increasingly used for energy metabolism during intensive training and competitive exertion, meaning autologous resources are affected, which are then no longer sufficiently available for the regeneration and stabilization of connective tissue. An insufficient micronutrient concentration along parameter PD/DPD, which is currently considered the best parameter for degenerative changes in bone and cartilage matrix, clearly shows the connection (see pg. 107-109).

Conclusion and evaluation

Every athlete who participated in this pilot project received individual training plans based on our biochemical functional analyses, for optimization of his personal performance, particularly in cases of existing muscular imbalances.

Video and detailed static analyses helped correct Initial misalignments or stresses.

Other risk factors were minimized at the start viaspecial dental exams and preventative measures in the area of microbiologic diagnostics. Our experience in recent years, while collaborating with the dental institute (Oberhofer & Partner Dentistry, Halle, Westphalia) shows definite connections between different injuries without external force.

Athletes with a good amino acid supply clearly exhibit fewer injuries without external force. Nutrition analyses conducted by nutritional scientists show a balanced diet and the positive effects of a simultaneous specific high-quality supplement of amino acids and other micronutrients.

An optimal supply of essential, but also to date nonessential amino acids, noticeably reduced injury risk. Athletes were given individual doses of an AM-formula blend and specifically prepared micronutrient formulations, using an add-on system based on the intracellular blood tests conducted by SALUTO Institute.

The recommendation made by many nutrition scientists and physicians to only supply selective whey protein powder in addition to a diet containing silica verifiably did not lead to replenishment of amino acids in the blood of 365 other athletes given 3-4 Tbsp per day, and thus does not show a reduced injury risk in these athletes.

Outlook

After preliminary special parameters (COMP, pyridine crosslink's in urine) and the results of increased injury risk in competitive athletes presented, we see a connection between cellular micronutrient deficiencies and degenerative changes in various connective tissue structures.

In the future we, along with our partners, will attempt to do detailed analyses of the effects of high-quality amino acids and other basic micronutrients on the injury-prone bradytrophic tissue structures of the tendon-ligament apparatus and cartilage structures in competitive athletes with the aid of modern MRT imaging and the special lab parameters shown.

Foto: Stockbyte

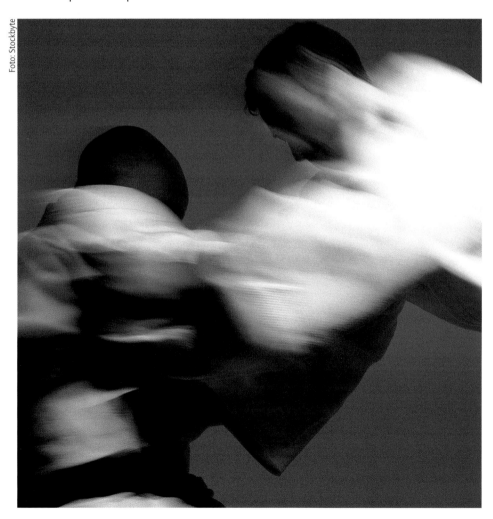

4.6 **Further research – newest lab parameters**

A pilot project with six triathletes from the Bundesliga, the first German League, (up to 25 hours training per week) over a period of four months (January through April) may suggest a preliminary trend. Along with very comprehensive immunological, special dental, biomechanical examinations and MRT imaging of the lumbar spine, knee joint, Achilles' tendon, one group received customized micronutrient formulations based on the respective athlete's cellular blood tests and at the same time up to 70 g of an AM-formula blend per day (given across the day).

The other group officially did not receive any micronutrients. Afterwards we heard from the athletes that supplements were also used in the other group, but due to differences in dosage no verifiable improvements of, for instance, the immune system (see pg. 126-128) could be seen. The nutrition analysis showed a balanced diet according to German Nutrition Society guidelines in all triathletes. The individual athletes' training logs were completed with the computer-assisted Polar analysis software.

The athletes' extensive and intensive training sessions verifiably led to increased metabolizing of autologous protein structures, resulting in their insufficient availability for basic connective tissue structures (tendons, ligaments, cartilage).

New parameters show links between degenerative changes in connective tissue structures and micronutrient deficiencies.

The newly developed special lab parameter COMP (see pg. 106) and the pyridine crosslinks in urine showed an initial clear connection between an optimal micronutrient formulation and avoidable inflammatory and degenerative changes in the triathletes. After four months, the triathletes with the customized micronutrient formulation showed clearly lower COMP levels than the group of triathletes that took micronutrient dosages based on German Nutrition Society guidelines.

> **Background information**
>
> As to the significance and use of the COMP (cartilage-oligometric-matrix-protein) parameter: Cartilage-oligometric-matrix-protein is a large extra-cellular matrix protein that occurs in cartilage, but also in other tissues, and whose function is largely unknown. Meanwhile this parameter is considered an indicator of increasing degenerative changes of various connective tissue structures (tendons, ligaments, cartilage).
>
> COMP occurs as an intact (pentrameric) protein, as an oligomeric as well as a monomeric fragment. When the joint cartilage breaks down due to injuries, degenerative or inflammatory processes, extra-cellular matrix matter increasingly gets into the synovial fluid and subsequently into the blood stream. The concentration of intact COMP as well as COMP fragments can be determined from serum with the aid of a sandwich ELISA. The biomarker is a specific and highly sensitive lab parameter for joint cartilage destruction in inflammatory and degenerative joint disorders such as rheumatoid arthritis or arthrosis, as well as acute trauma.

Contrary to other diagnostic methods (x-ray), COMP enables detection of possible joint damage and cartilage erosion already in the early stages and thus can be used reliably for risk assessment.

We measured this parameter in 200 competitive/top athletes. The COMP levels during a non-training phase initially were at 9.8 ± U/l. This level shows only a minor risk of possible degenerative changes in different connective tissue structures.

After two years, and a specific supply of customized micronutrient formulations in terms of the Anti-Doping-Concept (see pg. 169-170), unchanged COMP levels of 9.6 ± 1.3 U/l were measured in these 100 athletes.

The other athletes who had not received a specific supply of customized micronutrient formulations for two years initially showed unremarkable COMP levels of 10.1 ± 1.6 U/l. But after two years of intensive training and competition phases a definite increase in the level to 18.6 ± 2.6 U/l can be seen. This indicates increased degenerative changes in the stressed connective tissue structures. These athletes showed no evidence of recent knee trauma and torn ligaments that might have caused higher COMP levels.

Please note: There is no link between COMP concentrations and classic inflammation markers such as ESR (erythrocyte sedimentation rate) and CRP (C-reactive protein that can show possible inflammation). A one-time increase in the COMP level due to intensive athletic exertion was already discovered after a marathon in 1999. However, levels returned to normal after 24 hours (Neidhard et al, 2000).

Future tests will have to provide further proof as to the actual significance of this parameter with respect to degenerative changes in connective tissue structures. Tests with simultaneous MRT imaging after some years, will have to support these results.

Background information

Regarding the pyridinium crosslinks parameter: Our bones are subject to perpetual synthesis and breakdown. Bone synthesis occurs predominantly until approximately age 30 along with a constant increase in bone density. After that the course changes in direction of bone breakdown and at some point the breakdown process outweighs the synthesis process. Competitive athletes in particular often exhibit various injuries to the tendon-ligament apparatus and especially to cartilage structures that were previously never linked to a long-term insufficient supply of micronutrients.

Bone as well as cartilage consists of collagen molecules (see pg. 55-69) that are stabilized via crosslinks. In bone these crosslinks consist primarily of deoxypyridinoline (DPD), while in cartilage they are pyridinoline (PD). During intensified breakdown processes these crosslinks are released into the blood and subsequently eliminated in the urine. The amount of discharged pyridinium crosslinks depends on the degree of breakdown.

Since the exretions are neither impacted by neosynthesis of bone substance nor collagenous nutritional components, pyridinoline/deoxypiridiniura is currently considered the best marker to selectively identify possible degenerative changes in bone and cartilage substance.

Impact of an optimal micronutrient concentration on the PD/DPD parameter, the currently best indicator of increasing degenerative changes
(Connective tissue structures: cartilage/ bone substance in endurance athletes)

	Normal PD: DPD ratio < 4	DPD/crea target: 0-10 nmol/mmol creatinine	PD/crea target: 0-52 nmol/mmol creatinine
In 100 competitive athletes who will not receive customized micronutrient formulations, prior to the start of a training phase.	3.6 ± 0.33	8.3 ± 0.36	30 ± 3.8
In 100 competitive athletes who did not receive customized micronutrient formulations, after a two-year training/competition phase.	8.0 ± 0.41	18.1 ± 0.32	144.2 ± 7.3
In 100 competitive athletes who will subsequently receive customized micronutrient formulations, prior to the training phase.	3.7 ± 0.31	7.9 ± 0.27	29.4 ± 4.1
In 100 competitive athletes who did receive customized micronutrient formulations, after a two-year training/competition phase.	3.9 ± 0.40	9.3 ± 0.35	36.5 ± 6.1

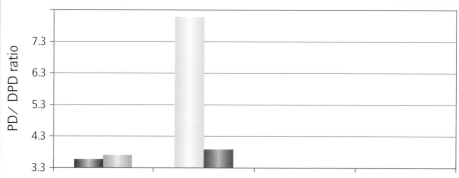

PD/ DPD ratio

Athletes without a customized micronutrient formulation, prior to the start of the training phase.

Athletes with a customized micronutrient formulation, prior to the start of the training phase.

Athletes without a customized micronutrient formulation, after the two-year training and competition phase.

Athletes with a customized micronutrient formulation, after the two-year training and competition phase.

Fig. 50

The results from pyridinium crosslinks confirm these results: The normal PD:DPD ratio is below four. A higher ratio with simultaneously high pyridinium levels indicates a higher breakdown rate of cartilage such as occurs in cases of rheumatoid arthritis. And that is precisely what we saw in the triathletes. Of the 559 competitive athletes (see pg. 101, 102) only 100 competitive athletes who had received a specific icustomized micronutrient formulation for two years, and had exhibited a verifiably decreased injury rate, had a normal PD:DPD ratio of 3.9 (nmol/mmol creatine). Deoxypyridinoline elimination was within a normal range. Competitive athletes who had not received a long-term customized micronutrient formulation showed a clearly higher ratio of 8.0 with simultaneously high pyridinium levels of 144.2 (nmol/mmol creatine). The analyses were done at the beginning and end of a three-day active regeneration phase.

The immune defense also benefitted from customized doses of micronutrients

The specific use of individually composed micronutrient formulations (vitamins, minerals, trace elements) and high-quality amino acids (AM-formula blend) lead to improved immune system activity (along the lines of the effects described on pg. 126-128), while the other group exhibited more frequent inflammation which then lead to brief training interruptions and thus did not permit optimal performance development.

In our experience, structural changes in the tendon-ligament apparatus and cartilage structures can be identified only after some years with the aid of MRT imaging (not, as previously thought, after 4-8 months).

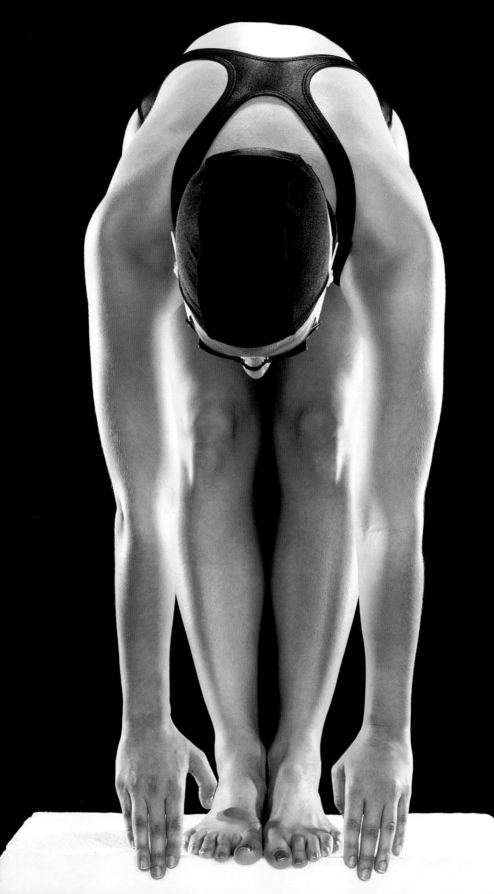

5   Prof. Dr. Elmar Wienecke's interview with Mark Warnecke

Author: Mr. Warnecke, the first time we met in person at SALUTO at the Gerry Weber Sportpark three years after you won the swimming world championships at age 35, I presented you with the test results from a total of 1,150 competitive athletes (see pg. 100-102). The competitive athletes from various disciplines that had received customized doses of micronutrient formulations and the AM-formula blend developed by you for a period of two years showed a significantly reduced injury rate compared to the athletes that had not received customized formulations. We have been successfully using the amino acid blend you developed with athletes for three years and have presented you with the results. Based on our experiences, considerably more qualitative protein (structural protein) is metabolized in the energy metabolism than previously thought (see pg. 82-89). In addition there are verifiably lower levels of other micronutrients in plants due to the described greenhouse effect (see pg. 40-43).

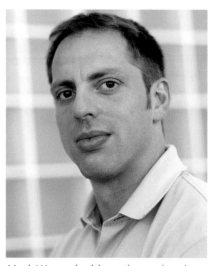

Mark Warnecke (three-time swimming world champion, ten-time German champion, oldest swimming world champion of all time at the age of 35, and current physician in private practice)

Question: As a physician, how do you explain the proven decrease in injury rates and thus the long-term training continuity of athletes who have received customized micronutrient formulations?

Mark Warnecke: That competitive athletes require more micronutrients has been known for a long time. The interesting test results you attained over the years show the verifiable connection between a sufficient micronutrient supply and a decrease in the injury rate in athletes. Competitive athletes live dangerously. Minor injuries to the connective tissue (ligaments, tendons, muscles) constantly prevent training continuity, not allowing the individual athlete to meet his performance potential. For competitive athletes an optimal supply of micronutrients is no longer possible in spite of a balanced diet. During intensive training and competition phases autologous structural proteins are metabolized, and thus are no longer sufficiently available as the organism's necessary "protective reserves" to keep the various connective tissue structures functioning. Injuries without external force are preprogrammed and thus diminish training continuity.

Author: We have previously attempted to show a link between degenerative changes in many connective tissue structures (tendon-ligament apparatus, but also different cartilage structures) and the long-term micronutrient deficiencies in triathletes, using expensive imaging methods. After the first four months a preliminary trend could be seen in the immune system, but no discernible change

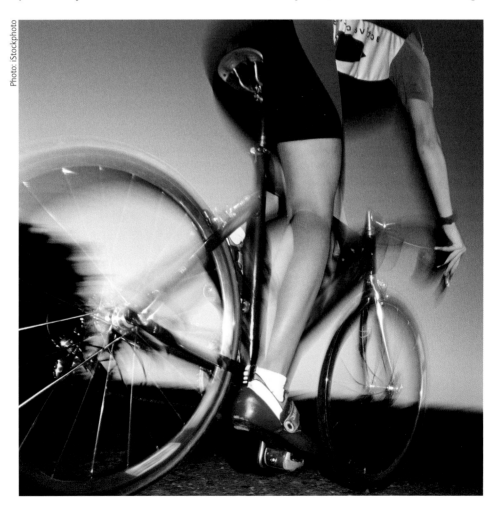

Photo: iStockphoto

in the tendon and ligament apparatus. The first specific tests with pyridinium crosslinks now show definite correlations. After lengthy discussions with radiologists and orthopedists we are of the opinion that such a verifiable effect can only be substantiated after several years through imaging techniques, and we intend to verify this connection with an innovative project. The results of the 559 competitive athletes who verifiably exhibit a negligible injury rate due to taking specific customized micronutrient formulations compared to the other group of 591 athletes, who did not receive customized micronutrient formulations but had a healthy diet (see pg.100-102), support our assumptions.

Question: What were your personal experiences with the specific use of micronutrients as an active athlete?

Mark Warnecke: For a top athlete specific substitution is absolutely necessary at a certain level of training. When I did Interval training on the bike in the midday sun, and even as a swimming sprinter rode just short of 40 km/h average in a 60 km/h unit, I needed primarily electrolytes and a quick resupply of fluids or I would have done damage to my body. The second biggest problem was of course a quick energy supply since I trained two to three times a day. Over the course of 15 years, I experimented with amino acids and learned to value their positive effects on metabolism and regeneration witha specific, sufficiently high dose.

Author: The high rate of injuries without external force in competitive recreational athletes and the blatant deficiencies of cellular micronutrient concentrations in 9,150 athletes in recent years show a direct link. It is exactly here that the application of new findings in the area of micronutrient therapy is urgently needed.

Question: In your opinion as a former top athlete, what is the situation for the average athlete?

Mark Warnecke: Based on your in-depth tests the average athlete is malnourished with respect to micronutrients, in spite of a diet improved by nutrition scientists. This sufficiently demonstrates the importance of a broad discussion on this topic. If there weren't so many people in official positions who shy away from responsibility out of ignorance, the research in this area could be advanced for the protection of athletes. Sports can do damage to athletes.

Ignorant statements such as "nutritional supplements don't do anything" only help the one who says it, because it is "in" to say so, although everyone should know that the candy bar after a workout when blood sugar is low, or the juice drink is nothing other than a type of nutritional supplement.

Author: Our experiences while spending time with 89 world champions, Olympic champions and European champions and 9,150 competitive athletes from many disciplines (German youth junior national team handball, soccer, track and field, martial arts) showed that these athletes exhibited an enormous cellular micronutrient deficiency and that the athletes who received specific customized micronutrient formulations experienced long-term replenishment of cellular micronutrient concentrations and thus training continuity.

Athletes live dangerously in the truest sense of the word if they train at the limit of their performance. The long-term heightened susceptibility to inflammation and the increased susceptibility to injury, particularly to connective tissue structures (tendon-ligament apparatus and many cartilage structures), can verifiably be reduced with the specific use of cusotmized micronutrient formulations without any banned substances.

Question: Elite sports without banned substances are still possible. Maybe the cyclists in the Tour de France ride a little slower, but with customized micronutrient formulations they will be healthier. As a former successful competitive athlete and current physician, what is your personal opinion?

Mark Warnecke: Elite sports without banned substances are still possible and will continue to be. However, we physicians need to act on your research results and dispense specific customized micronutrient formulations to competitive athletes to allow them to definitely reduce their injury risk long-term and boost their performance potential.

Author: These days you are being sneered at by some of your medical colleagues who accuse you of just wanting to sell your products. What would you say to those critics? A scientific analysis of athletes conducted at the 2004 Olympics in Athens concluded that based on the existing results a need for general substitution in top athletes did not exist.

Mark Warnecke: As was previously mentioned, no competitive athlete can do without the specific customized micronutrient formulations you described. During neutral testing the amino acid blend I developed as an athlete and physician proved to be effective in clearly lowering the risk of injury. This also coincides with my own experiences as an athlete.

I will continue to conduct other research projects in the future that will surely confirm this evidence. My personal concern will continue to be permanent advancement. The development of an amino acid blend is the result of a lot of meticulous work and its proven success in the maintenance of connective tissue function through your research results pleases me immensely.

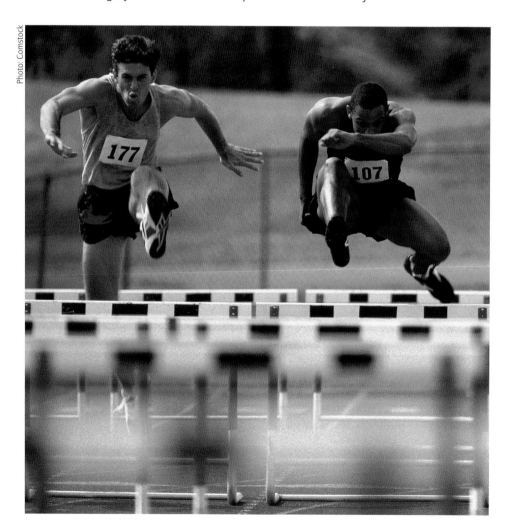

Photo: Comstock

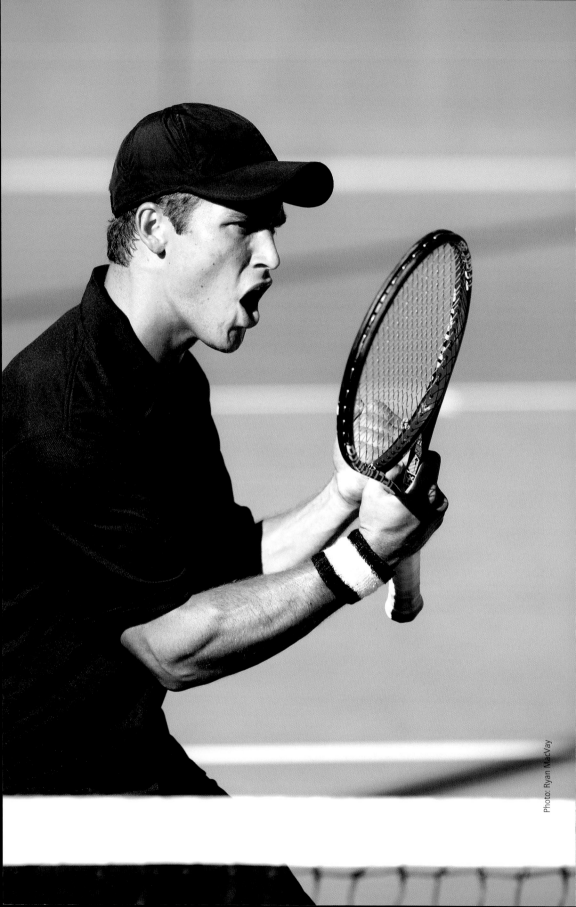

6   Sports and the immune system – a balancing act for competitive athletes

6.1   General aspects

Every minute of our life our body is exposed to many damaging agents, including radiation, toxins and microorganisms such as bacteria or viruses. In addition there are diseased or abnormal autologous cells. It therefore possesses defense mechanisms to protect it. An important part of the defense mechanism is the *lymphatic* system. The body fluid it transports, the *lymph*, is high in lymphocytes and proteins and is very similar to plasma.

The lymphocytes produce antibodies and activate the immune system. Lymphocytes accumulate in the so-called *lymph nodes*. In the event of an infection their activity increases, they multiply and are increasingly released into the bloodstream, externally visible by swollen lymph nodes (glands). Furthermore, the lymphatic vessels transport substances that should not, or rather cannot reach the bloodstream. Such substances are for instance dietary fats and particles that are unable to penetrate the capillary walls, such as bacteria and tumor cells.

The body formed a number of defense mechanisms prior to birth that will provide non-specific protection form these threats. This resistance to pathogens or their toxins is due to natural safeguards like the epidermis and mucous membranes, and cellular defense from certain "defense cells". The body's resistance can be lowered by external factors such as exhaustion, malnutrition or undernourishment, stress, etc. In addition to the non-specific innate immunity the body also has acquired immunity. This process extends from the identification of a penetrating antigen, its phagocytosis, the forming of antibodies, to the destruction of the antigen or its toleration by autologous antigens.

Each antigen intrusion (bacteria, viruses, etc.) triggers a threefold process:

1. There is an increase in the forming of macroglobulin in the blood serum, which attaches itself to the foreign proteins.

2. Specific antibodies are formed to neutralize the antigens.

3. Thymus lymphocytes increase.

Immune defense can essentially be classified based on its function and acquisition. The transitions from specific to non-specific immune system are fluid and cannot be viewed as separate. Here we only describe the parameters of lymphocyte differentiation (T-lymphocytes, B-lymphocytes, T-helper cells, phagocytosis activity). Due to cost requirements we abandoned further testing of different interleukins.

This table shows the many non-specific and specific aspects of immunity:

Table 6: Aspects of specific and nonspecific immunity

	Nonspecific immune system	Specific immune system
	Susceptibility does not decrease with repeated infection.	Susceptibility decreases with repeated infection.
Soluble (humoral) factors	Complement, lysozyme, interferon	Antibodies (immunoglobuline) are released via B-lymphocytes.
Cell-mediated (cellular) immunity	Phagocytes, natural killer cells	T-lymphocytes • Helper cells • Cytotoxic cells

Innate or non-specific defense

The non-specific or innate immunity developed very early on in life's phylogeny. It includes anatomical and physiological barriers like epithelia but also cell-mediated resistance via phagocytosis, as well as generally inflammatory reactions and the complement system. Ordinarily foreign germs do not easily penetrate the uppermost dermal layers and the prevalent pH-value in that area (slightly acidic) makes it difficult for them to enter the body.

If a microorganism does manage to overcome the epithelial barrier, it is immediately attacked by different molecules as well as special cells, the macrophages, natural killer cells and neutrophil granulocytes, that recognize it via germline-encoded receptors and are able to distinguish it from autologous cells. The innate immunity can thereby fight pathogens without previous direct contact between the organism and the germ.

These special innate immunity receptors include for instance the so-called *toll-like receptors* (TLR) that can recognize pathogenic microorganisms. TLR's only recognize pathogens that are located outside the cell or in the endosomes. For that reason localized cytosolic receptors, for example RIG-I (retinoic acid inducible gene I) that can recognize reproducing viruses by the peculiarities of their ribonucleic acid, play an important role. In doing so the immune system uses unchanging characteristics of the pathogens, the so-called *pathogen-associated molecular patterns* (PAMP). These are so closely linked to the germ's survival and/or pathogenic characteristics that it cannot easily change them to perhaps avoid the immune reaction. With respect to TLR's, the term "non-specific" immune defense leads to a misconception since the recognition of PAMP's is a very specific function. That is why the term *bow-tie architecture* was coined with respect to TLR's: A limited number of receptors recognize many microbial structures via a few specific core motifs.

Macrophages and neutrophil granulocytes contain *inflammasome*, a protein complex that is stimulated by parts of bacteria or uric acid crystals. This prompts a series of reactions that finally lead to the activation of the proinflammatory cytokine interleukin 1ß. This is excreted by the macrophages and triggers the inflammatory response. If bacteria activated the inflammsome, the inflammatory response plays an important role in the defense against the infection. However, if uric acid crystals triggered the infection it will result in a gout attack.

In addition the innate immune defense is also able to distinguish autologous cells from foreign structures. For this purpose practically every cell in the body has access to the so-called major *histocompatibility complex* (MHC) which is basically the cell's "membership pass". Exogenous or diseased cells without access to MHC are thereby identified and inevitably become the target of a defense action.

90% of all infections are identified by the innate immune defense

It is assumed that approximately 90% of all infections can be identified and successfully fought via the innate immune defense. These defense strategies were therefore adopted nearly unchanged in the course of phylogenetic development of basic life forms to complex organisms. For instance, a comparison between the immune defense of insects and the innate portion of the human immune defense reveals many similarities.

Different cells carry out the duties of the innate immune defense. Next to the previously mentioned cell types these also include eosinophilic granulocytes, basophilic granulocytes, dentritic cells and epithelial cells. These cells are to some extent capable of destroying the attacker (germ) themselves. In addition they put the organism into a state of alert by producing messengers (interleukin) and thus are able to amplify the immune reaction. The effect of some of these messengers can be recognizedby, for instance, inflammation and fever.

Adaptive or specific defense

The *specific* or *adaptive immune* defense, formerly also referred to as *acquired immune system*, developed from the innate immune defensein the course of vertebrate phylogeny. It distinguishes itself by its adaptability as compared to new or modified pathogens. Within the bounds of this adaptation the cells of the adaptive immune defense are capable of identifying the attackers' specific structures (antigens) and selectively forming cellular defense mechanisms and molecular antibodies.

Next to antigen-presenting cells (APC) like dendritic cells, two groups of cells make up the integral adaptive immunity elements. The T-lymphocytes, which on the one hand provide the cell-mediated immune response and on the other hand support the B-lymphocytes, as well as the lymphocytes themselves which are responsible for the humoral immunity, meaning for those methods of defense that are directed against invaders in bodily fluids (humors) via secreted antibodies. After the infection specific antibodies and memory cells remain intact to quickly facilitate an appropriate response upon renewed contact with the pathogen.

However, the adaptive immune system does not replace the innate one but rather cooperates with it. The various parts of the immune system are mutually dependent. Only a well-coordinated interplay between innate and adaptive immune defense makes the body's complex immune response possible.

Short-term effects of
intensive athletic exertion on the immune system

Any athletic exertion causes an inflammation-like response. As long as athletic exertion is moderate the "radio traffic" of many immune system structures improves. But during long-term intensive and extensive training and competition phases the risk of infection clearly increases. At the same time cellular micronutrient concentrations clearly decrease and show considerable deficiencies. Our results show a direct link between a targeted individual supply of micronutrients in athletes and a reduced risk of infection, particularly in the upper respiratory area.

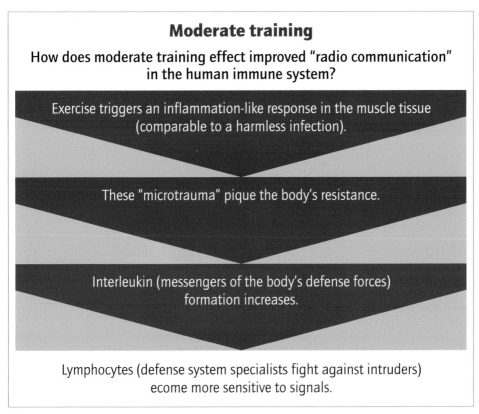

Moderate training

How does moderate training effect improved "radio communication" in the human immune system?

Exercise triggers an inflammation-like response in the muscle tissue (comparable to a harmless infection).

These "microtrauma" pique the body's resistance.

Interleukin (messengers of the body's defense forces) formation increases.

Lymphocytes (defense system specialists fight against intruders) ecome more sensitive to signals.

Fig. 51

6.2   Components of the immune system

The various components of the immune system are:

- mechanical barriers to prevent penetration by germs,

- cells such as the granulocytes, natural killer cells (NK cells) or T-lymphocytes. Some are combined into specialized organs (lymphatic system);

- Proteins that serve as messengers or as defense against pathogens and

- psychological factors.

Mechanical and physiological barriers

The body's mechanical and physiological barriers are the first line of defense against pathogens. They make sure that the pathogens are unable to penetrate the body or leave it again as quickly as possible:

- Skin – outer layer serves as barrier; sebum, sweat and normal flora as impediments to growth of pathogenic microorganisms;

- Mucous membrane – mucous binding;

- Eyes – tear evacuation, antimicrobial enzyme lysozyme fights microorganisms;

- Respiratory tracts – mucous binding, evacuation of cilia;

- Oral cavity – antimicrobial enzyme lysozyme in the saliva fights microorganisms;

- Stomach – stomach acid (containing hydrochloric acid) and enzymes that break down proteins destroy nearly all bacteria and microorganisms;

- Intestines – bacteria (intestinal flora) provide infection defense, evacuation via constant emptying and the so-called *intestinal immune system* (GALT = gut-associated lymphoid tissue) and bacterial proteins, and the

- urinary tract – evacuation via constant urinary washout as well as osmotic effects of high urea concentration.

Components of a cell

The cells of the immune system circulate in the blood vessels and lymph channels and occur in the body's tissue. If a pathogen enters the body the defense cells are able to fight it. Neutrophil granulocytes, monocytes/macrophages and dentritic cells can destroy the pathogen via absorption and digestion (phagocytosis), or control the organism's immune response with the production of immune modulators and cytokines and attract other defense cells to the inflammation site.

Granulocytes

Granulocytes (lat. granulum: granule) make up the bulk of the white blood cells (leucocytes). They can leave the bloodstream and migrate into the tissue. Granulocytes have many vesicles in the cytoplasm containing aggressive subs-tances that can render the pathogens innocuous. Other substances (for instance histamine) also play a role in the inflammatory response and allergies. The different granulocyte groups are classified based on their staining reaction within the Giemsa staining protocol.

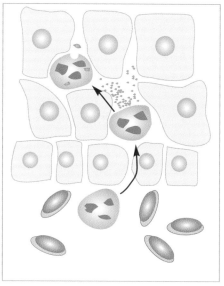

Fig. 52: A neutrophil granulocyte migrates from the blood vessel to the tissue, secretes proteolytic enzymes to dissolve intercellular connections (to improve mobility) and engulfs and destroys bacteria.

- The *neutrophil* granulocytes make up 40-50% of the circulating leucocytes. Activated by cytokines that are secreted from the in-flammation site, they migrate from the blood vessels to the effected tissue. The neutrophil granules contain, among other things, acid hydrola, defensin (30% of content), myeloperoxidase and protease, such as elastase, collagenase, neuraminidase and cathepsin g. This "cocktail" enables the neutrophil to channel through the tissue and reach the bacteria. There they are able to destroy pathogens (for instance bacteria) by, among others, phagocytosis.

- *Eosinophile* granulocytes make up 3-5% of the cells in the differential blood count. They derive their name from the stain *eosin*, with which they can be colored. Eosinophils are also capable of *chemotaxis*, meaning they can move towards an inflammation site. Eosinophils contain basic proteins in their granules, such as the major basic protein, which they can release after stimulation from class igE antibodies. Eosinophils play an important role in parasite defense. A parasite infestation therefore results in a large increase of eosinophils in the blood. The number of eosinophils also increases with allergies, which indicates that eosinophils are not beneficial to this illness either.

- *Basophile* granulocytes possess numerous rough, uneven granules that contain, among other things, histamine and heparine. They make up only a small portion (< 2%) of the differential blood count. When their receptors are stimulated by allergen-bound IgE basophiles, they release toxic mediators like histamine and the platelet-activating factor (PAF). However, the physiological significance of basophiles is largely unclear.

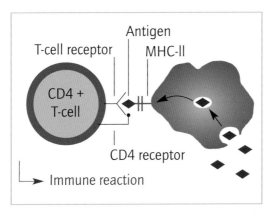

Fig. 53: A macrophage engulfs an antigen in order to present it to a T-helper cell via its MHC class II complex. The T-cell subsequently initiates the immune response.

Macrophages

Macrophages (Giant phagocytes) also constitute a portion of the immune system. Macrophages mature from monocytes (mono-nuclear white blood cells = mononuclear leucocytes) that leave the bloodstream. Macrophages reside in the tissue where they identify and devour (phagocytosis) invading pathogens. If the macrophages are not able to fight the pathogens they can activate the adaptive immune defense. To this end the engulfed parts of the pathogen are broken down into individual peptides (epitopes) inside the macrophages and presented on the surface via MHC class II molecules. Thus macrophages turn into antigen-presenting cells. T-helper cells identify antigens in this way and subsequently initiate an adaptive immune response that finally leads to the pathogen's destruction. Macrophages also play a major role in the fight against and the elimination of harmful substances and waste products (e.g. tar from cigarette smoke in the lungs) which is why it is occasionally referred to as "the body's garbage disposal".

6.3 The specific use of micronutrients and their impact on the immune system

Determining the effects of targeted use of micronutrients on the immune system is extremely complex. These micronutrients are not the standard dosages of multivitamins, but rather formulations that are only available through pharmacies and can be composed with a modular system based on cellular analyses of vital substances. Next to the customized formulations the athletes received AM formula-blend in doses determined for each individual. In addition the blood analysis results of the complex immune system must meet certain prerequisites to be accurately interpreted.

These special, very elaborate and expensive blood tests of portions of the specific and non-specific immunity should be completed prior to a preparatory or competitive phase (four days without training, apart from regeneration). Otherwise the preceding intensive exertion will affect certain immune system reactions.

In addition bacterial or viral infections should be excluded from the interpretation of results.

New research plans

We previously gave a detailed description of the positive effects of a specific customized micronutrient formulation on injury risk. Our initial test results with pyridinium-Crosslinks (see pg. 107, 108) imaging show the link between long-term micronutrient deficiencies and the degeneration of many connective tissue structures. In the foreseeable future, we will conduct a large-scale research project with competitive athletes over a period of many years, to ultimately be able to corroborate the previous results with empirical scientific data.

How we tested

We had a pharmacist prepare a specific customized micronutrient formulation for a total of 123 soccer players from a German Regional League team for a period of five months. The formulation was taken in the morning and with lunch. In addition the players were dosed with 30 to 60 grams of an AM-formula blend (high-quality amino acids) distributed throughout the day).

Another group of players (N = 113) did not receive a customized micronutrient supply. In some cases standard doses of multivitamin preparations were being used. The players did not train for four days prior to the beginning and exit examinations.

Blood test results

The blood test results showed a statistically significant rise in T-lymphocytes, B-lymphocytes and T-helper cells in the players that had received a specific customized micronutrient supply. There were no discernible changes of immunological parameters in the control group.

Only players without bacterial or viral infections at the time of testing were included. An increase in these immunological factors always indicates an improved cellular specific and non-specific immunity in some parts.

However, cell cycles must be within a normal range before and after the five-month period. The future will reveal to what extend the rise in T-lymphocytes and T-helper cells in the peripheral blood is responsible for the decreased susceptibility to infection. Measuring of the different cytokines In particular would be useful. Here, too, additional positive effects might be detected via LTT (lymphocyte transformation test) or rather the determination of TH-1 and TH-2 cytokines.

Phagocytic activity of monocytes and granulocytes as an indicator of nonspecific immunity also increased significantly in the group of players with a specific customized supply of micronutrients. However, the fluctuation range of the measurement can be relatively large (up to 20%).

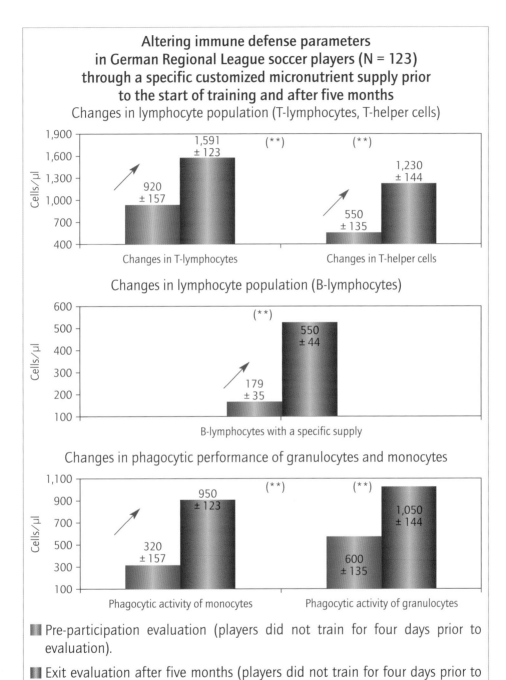

Altering immune defense parameters
in German Regional League soccer players (N = 123)
through a specific customized micronutrient supply prior
to the start of training and after five months

Changes in lymphocyte population (T-lymphocytes, T-helper cells)

Changes in lymphocyte population (B-lymphocytes)

Changes in phagocytic performance of granulocytes and monocytes

■ Pre-participation evaluation (players did not train for four days prior to evaluation).

■ Exit evaluation after five months (players did not train for four days prior to evaluation).

Bacterial or viral infections at the time of the evaluations can be ruled out.

Fig. 54

127

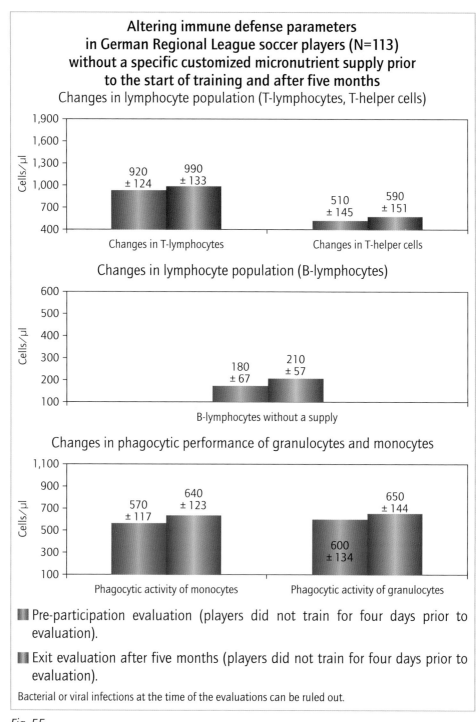

Fig. 55

Conclusion: The group of players with a specific customized micronutrient supply had nearly no downtime due to infection (4.3%) during the test period. In the other group of 113 players 53% experienced downtime.

An important factor (see box): all players were given a positive dental health status prior to our tests by means of special concomitant dental exams and preventative treatment based on those results.

Impact of dental health status on the immune system

Within the scope of the unique European prevention program with German youth and junior national level team handball players we, along with our partners (Oberhofer & Partner Dentistry), found a direct link between the players' dental health status and their immune system.

After extremely cost-intensive examinations (microbiological analyses of existing germs) and additional comprehensive dental diagnostics with an intraoral camera, the players were able to take the specific results with them with the intent to correct existing problems and perform preventative measures. These included specific use of dental floss and interdental brushes. In addition players were asked to have their teeth cleaned twice a year by a certified dental hygienist.

The effects of inadequate oral hygiene (e.g. initial signs of gingivitis) and/or the presence of pathogenic germs can have a verifiably negative effect on the nonspecific immune system. We will forgo a detailed description.

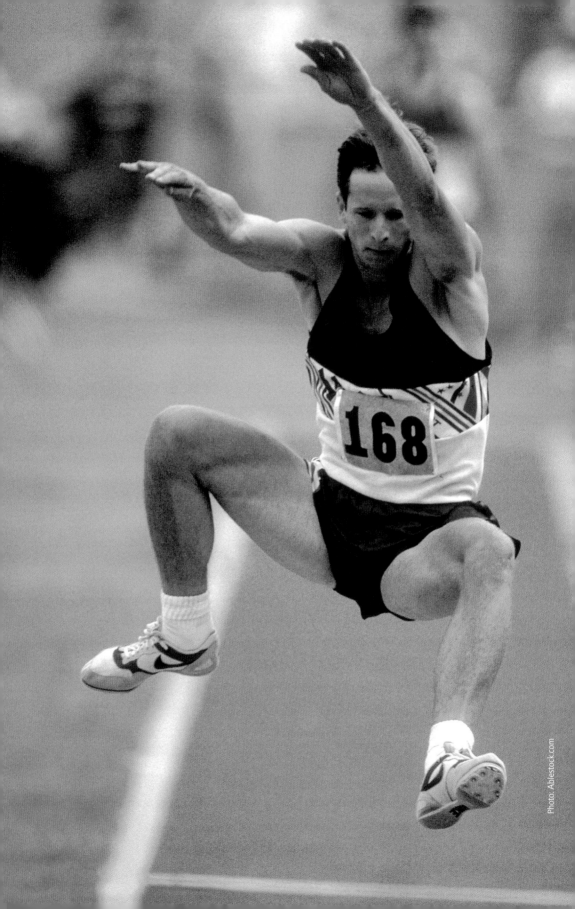

7 Important tasks of individual micronutrients

This is an introduction to some of the micronutrients that are particularly important to active athletes. We will forgo a complete description of tasks, occurrence and functions of vitamins, minerals and trace elements and the respective reference values of blood tests, but will refer to the table "Dosage recommendations for micronutrients in recreational and competitive athletes in terms of customized micronutrient formulations", see pg. 171, 172.

7.1 Optimal iron supply – ensuring performance

As a fundamental building block of the red blood pigment hemoglobin, iron is essential for the transport of oxygen in blood and the oxygen supply in the cellular energy metabolism (in the mitochondria = "cellular powerhouse"). A good iron supply is indispensible to optimal mental and physical performance and immune function. Our muscle cells cannot produce energy without oxygen.

Iron deficiency is the most frequently diagnosed mineral deficiency in sports medicine. The athlete feels tired and sluggish and does not sufficiently regenerate after intensive training.

Symptoms of iron deficiency include:

*   decreased performance,

*   general fatigue,

*   anemia,

*   lacerations at the corners of the mouth

*   impaired hair and nail growth.

Due to increased iron loss in sweat and urine via the gastro-intestinal tract, athletes have higher iron requirements that are not always met by a balanced diet containing meat. Next to vegetarian athletes, athletes with an increased risk of developing an iron deficiency are female endurance athletes, as well as adolescent male and female athletes due to menses and growth-related factors. Long distance runners in particular develop iron deficiencies primarily through perspiration (0.3-0.7 mg/l) and exertion-related blood loss in the gastro-intestinal tract (1 ml of blood contains 0.5 mg of iron).

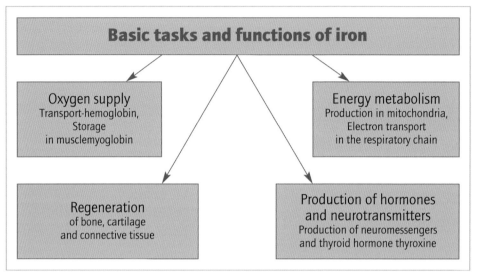

Fig. 56

Assessing iron status

Assessing iron in serum is not a suitable diagnosis for iron deficiency. Since the ferritin level in serum correlates well with tissue iron, this test is considered standard. An iron deficiency exists when the serum ferritin level is 1µg/l (equals approximately 8-10 mg storage iron). For athletes regularly scheduled iron assessments are indispensible.

In women serum ferritin levels of < 40 are already associated with diffuse hair loss. Ferritin levels in endurance athletes should be at the following levels to achieve optimal endurance capacity:

Women: athletic women > 60 ng/ml

Men: athletic men > 80 ng/ml

> **Important information**
>
> Elevated CrP levels (acute phase protein) and a possible increase in leucocytes (white blood cells) can affect the ferritin count. Please take this into account when interpreting the results.

There is some controversy regarding the optimal ferritin level. This reference data is based on our experience with 9,150 athletes and studies we conducted.

High iron storage (serum ferritin > 200 µg/l) is linked to higher risk of chronic degenerative disorders and a higher cancer risk. Oxidative stress may play a central role. The more non-oxidized iron reaches the large intestine the higher the exposure to free radicals, which can result in damage to the mucous membrane.

> **Important information**
>
> A targeted iron supply should only be taken after a lab diagnostic test. Taking a high dose of iron (e.g. 50-100 mg/day) without doctor's advice is not recommended. Random use of too much iron can increase exposure to free radicals and requires previous accurate diagnostics.

Recommendations for supplementing iron based on lab tests

Recommended supply of divalent iron taken orally: long-term regular use of low doses of iron (e.g. 60 mg/day) is more sensible since high doses of iron supplements can frequently cause gastrointestinal upset (e.g. diarrhea, nausea, constipation). But this can be determined individually in particular cases. We had good results with athletes who had low ferritin levels < 40 µg/ml taking *ferro sanol duodenal*® once daily in the evening with food for a four-week period. After four weeks the iron supply was continued 2-3 times per week until the next blood test (circa 6-8 weeks).

Important: Next to per os iron supplements (divalent iron), in cases of poor iron statusit may be wise to initially do an iron infusion therapy (trivalent iron) to compensate the iron deficiency relatively quickly. The dosage depends on the level of iron deficiency (e.g. 50-100 mg iron (III) hydroxide/dextran in 0.9% NaCl, two to three times per week, slow I.V.) Prior to the infusion 25 mg of iron should be administered over a period of 15 minutes.

A ferritin deficiency (iron storage form) can exist even with a good hemoglobin concentration. Additional methods to assess iron status are: transferring saturation ("iron transport"), soluble transferring receptor, volume and hemoglobin concentration of erythrocytes (red blood cells).

Important information

Caution must be used when taking iron supplements: Ideally these should be taken on an empty stomach 0,5 to 1 hour before a meal. In our experience many athletes have frequent problems with taking iron supplements. In that case we recommend taking it with food. Orange juice (vitamin C) stabilizes the oxidation-sensitive iron and improves resorption. Iron is used primarily in the form of iron (II) gluconate and iron (II) fumarate.

Iron deficiency limits endurance capacity

We examined a total of four groups of female athletes who, over a period of three months, completed a specified endurance workout based on our physical performance assessments four times a week for 60 minutes. It was recommended to half the athletes, due to low ferritin levels (women < 40 ng/ml, men < 60 ng/ml), to take *ferro sanol duodenal®* (active ingredient iron (II) glycine sulfate complex) in the evenings with food for the first month.

Due to deficient intracellular magnesium concentrations all participants received additional *magnerot classic®* chewable tablets, 3 x 35 mg morning and afternoon. As is known, magnesium and iron compete with each other for absorption. The test subjects therefore received *ferro sanol duodenal®* in the evenings with food (due to better tolerability).

After one month, the athletes took iron only three times per week in the evenings since a daily long-term medication containing iron can have a negative effect on the immune system. All test subjects had already mentioned some fatigue at the start of the project. The nutritional analysis showed that the athletes had a balanced diet as per DGE (German Nutrition Society) guidelines.

Impact of a specific supply of iron on the development of endurance capacity in male and female athletes				
	Female athletes		Male athletes	
	Control group	Specific iron supply	Control group	Specific iron supply
Number	102	115	94	98
Age (years)	21.3 ± 3.2	24.3 ± 4.8	24.3 ± 3.9	26.8 ± 4.8
BMI (kg/m²)	23.7 ± 1.5	21.1 ± 1.9	23.2 ± 1.5	24.3 ± 1.7

Fig. 57

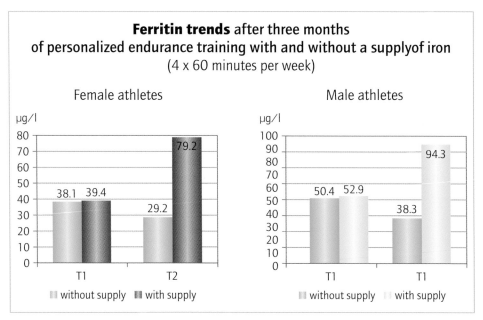

Fig. 58

Our test results

Our test results show the importance of an optimal iron supply for the development of endurance capacity. The already low ferritin levels in athletes who did not receive a specific iron supply decreased even after the three-month training phase. These athletes described increasing fatigue that was manifested by a certain listlessness.

The two illustrations show that the development of endurance capacity (measured with individual aerobic and anaerobic threshold and fixed threshold at 4 mmol/l) in the athletes with the specific iron supply led to a statistically most significantly

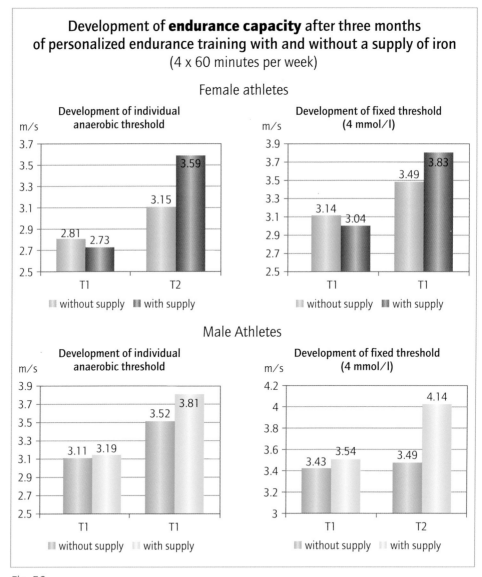

Fig. 59

higher increase compared to the athletes with the ferritin deficiencies that had been determined at the onset. Please note that the speciifc iron supply can only be administered after a previous blood test.

Nutrition tips for a diet rich in iron

The body utilizes iron obtained from animal products (fish, meat) two times better than iron from plant products. For that reason endurance athletes should only forgo meat and fish if they consume corresponding amounts of ferrous plant foods. Aiding as well as inhibiting factors of iron intake must also be taken into consideration.

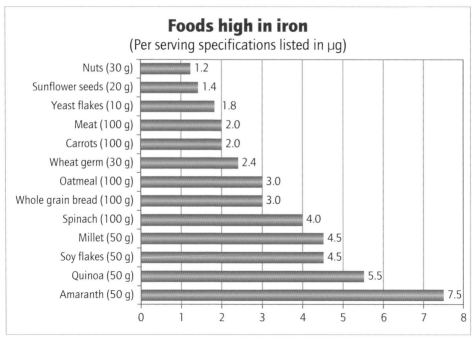

Fig. 60: Compiled from DGE nutrition panel, 43rd edition, 2005

Iron from plant sources

•   Amaranth is a cultivated plant. Amaranth is one of humanity's oldest agricultural crops. It is used primarily for its millet-like seeds. Even the Aztec, Inca and Maya used its grain (amaranthus caudatus, predominantly called kiwicha; in the Andes regionthis name is stillused today) as a staple food next to quinoa and corn. Amaranth is one of the few plants containing qualitative carbohydrates, protein and minerals. It can be cooked like rice or can be sprinkled over cereal in the form of amaranth pops. The grains can be purchased in natural food stores.

- A suggestion for iron in salads: Lightly toast 2 Tbs sunflower seeds per person in a skillet without fat. Sprinkle toasted sunflower seeds over salad.

- Spinach as a source of iron is overrated. Unfortunately previous recommendations on spinach consumption were based on an analytical error. Please forgo eating spinach several times each week since spinach contains oxalic acid, which can have a negative effect on calcium absorption.

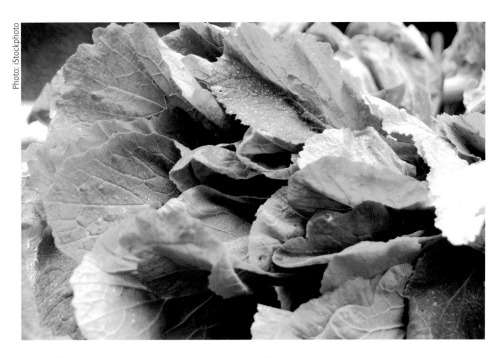

Photo: iStockphoto

What boosts or inhibits iron absorption

Facilitators of good iron absorption:

- sprouts in salads

- vitamin C with food (orange juice, fruit, fresh bell peppers) and

- lactic acid in whey, yoghurt, Sauerkraut.

Eat these foods regularly. Endurance athletes should regularly eat germinated grains because bioavailability in sprouts is excellent due to the germination process.

Factors that may inhibit iron absorption:

• phytic acid

• phosphate and

• tannic acid (black/green tea, coffee).

Avoid foods or beverages that are high in phosphates. Colas are particularly high in phosphates. Their consumption should be limited. If it is difficult to abstain from its consumption, it should at least not be consumed with meals.

Drinking coffee or tea

An athlete doesn't have to deny himself the occasional cup of coffee. Athletes who enjoy drinking coffee do not have to give it up.

Please allow a period of time between drinking coffee and a healthy athlete's breakfast, e.g. with wheat germ or amaranth pops. This facilitates better iron absorption by the gastrointestinal tract.

Green or black tea contains a lot of tannic acid, and the longer it steeps the more there is. For this reason tea should not be allowed to steep longer than 1-2 minutes. Coffee also contains tannic acid. An athlete who drinks coffee should get used to drinking only one cup after a meal, rather than three cups. Coffee inhibits iron absorption only if consumed in high volume (4-5 cups a day).

Two more tips:

• If you tolerate coffee well, drinking two cups of coffee before a competition is recommended to elevate excitement, alertness and mindset. Higher doses can lead to nervousness, which will have a negative effect.

• **Caution:** coffee has a diuretic effect. For this reason athletes should forgo coffee consumption during long competitions to avoid additional impact on the body's fluid balance.

7.2 Magnesium – the do-all of minerals

Magnesium is involved in more than 300 enzymatic processes. These are directly linked to the energy storage substance ATP (adenosine triphosphate). Magnesium plays a central role in muscle contraction, impulse transmission in nerve and muscle cells, the stabilization of cell membranes and the control of heart muscle function. A sufficient supply increases stress resistance and prevents rapid exhaustion of the cellular energy repository and electrolytes.

A magnesium deficiency increases the permeability to potassium, which interferes with cellular potassium replenishment and has a negative effect on physical performance and heartbeat frequency. The calcium's antagonistic effect on magnesium protects the heart muscle from calcium overload. Thus magnesium economizes the heart muscle's bioenergetics, particularly during high stress, and prevents arrhythmia.

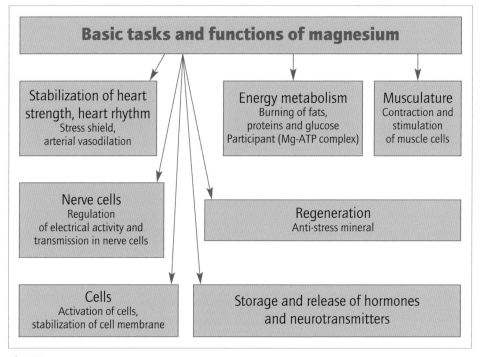

Fig. 61

Magnesium deficiency is one of the most common mineral deficiencies in athletes

Typical symptoms of magnesium deficiency include:

- premature fatigue,

- muscle weakness,

- weak muscle response

- tendency to painful muscle and calf cramps,

- muscle hardening,

- eyelid twitching and

- decline in regeneration and training adaptation.

Different studies show a magnesium deficiency of more than 65% (see Saur, 2004).

Measuring intraerythrocyte levels would be particularly wise (diagnostics, see pg. 34-40, 50, Fig. 26). Our own studies, as well as those of others, have shown that there are considerable gaps in the assessment of mineral status in serum and plasma since there is no correlation between serum concentration and the concentration in blood cells (red blood cells) (see Saur, 2004). The results from our clinical study show a statistically significant increase in the magnesium concentration while the cellular concentration decreases.

Conclusion: The "status quo" of the magnesium balance can only be accurately assessed with the aid of special cellular blood tests.

Depletion of Intracellular magnesium in particular can lead to a diminished athletic performance. Approximately 80% of cellular ATP's are complex-bound to magnesium. Magnesium loses its bonding partner when ATP is fused due to physical exertion. This results in an intracellular release of magnesium and a deficit in tissues. The shift from intra to extracellular space can cause magnesium levels to be temporarily deceptively high in spite of the deficit. The kidneys react to the high magnesium level with increased elimination, thus increasing magnesium depletion.

Dosage recommendations for magnesium

An optimal cellular magnesium concentration in competitive athletes can only be achieved with special diagnostics. Cellular deficiencies require long-term use of magnesium. Short-term use of 4-6 weeks cannot replenish cellular stores.

Competitive athletes with major cellular deficiencies (< 40 mg/l ery.) should initially undergo intravenous magnesium therapy under a doctor's supervision, accompanied by a regular orally administered magnesium supply. Dosage should be between 2.048-4.095 mg $MgSO_4$(=201.9-403.8 = 8.3-16.6.mmol/l) slow IV, for instance 2-3 times a week for three weeks.

Optimal supplements due to their availability are magnesium preparations with organic magnesium salts such as magnesium orotate, taurate, citrate, gluconate and aspartate. We have had exceedingly good results with *magnerot classic®*, 3 x 35 mg chewable tablets. The positive effects of magnesium orotate on athletic performance appear to be caused by the synergistic effects of magnesium and orotic acid. Both substances have an activating effect on the metabolism, particularly the energy metabolism. Orotic acid also facilitates magnesium fixation and thus can counteract performance-limiting magnesium loss.

Dosage recommendations: For example, for recreational athletes doing up to four hours of endurance training, *magnerot classic®* 3 x 35 mg in the morning and 3 x 35 mg in the evening in the form of chewable tablets taken with food. For more intensive training, 3 x 35 mg in the morning, afternoon and evening in the form of chewable tablets.

Ideal would be a magnesium preparation without sweeteners or other additives. These can easily cause gastrointestinal upset (e.g. diarrhea).

The effect of an optimal magnesium supply on endurance capacity

In many of the studies we conducted ourselves we were able to find a direct relationship to an optimal cellular magnesium concentration. During a three-month training phase 48 athletes did not receive any magnesium supplements while a group of 52 athletes took *magnerot classic*® 35 mg chewable tablets in the morning, afternoon and evening with food (dosage according to measured magnesium concentration).

Ferritin levels in both groups of examined athletes showed a sufficient iron supplyof 80.9 ± 8.9. The endurance capacity of athletes with a cellular magnesium concentration of < 44 mg/l ery. measured against the fixed threshold, improved only 9.1% at 4 mmol/l ery. (from 3.70 ± 0.30 to 4.07 ± 0.12), while the athletes with a magnesium concentration of > 55 mg/l ery., were able to improve upon the fixed threshold by 14.7% (from 3.81 ± 0.19 to 4.47 ± 0.11). The training volume was the same for both groups. This clearly shows the significance of this parameter to the development of endurance capacity.

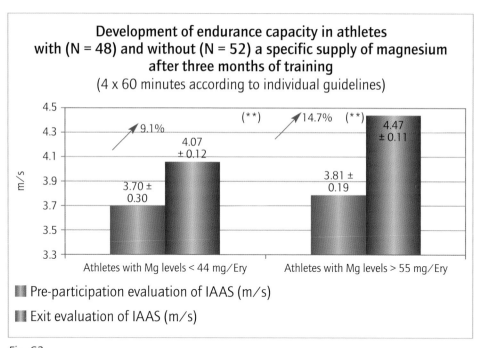

Fig. 62

Along the lines of this study, the 1994 Gießen triathlon study (Geiss et al, 1994) showed similar results. In a double blind, randomized study 23 triathletes received either magnesium orotate or placebos for a period of three months. The group with the specific magnesium supplement was able to increase its performance by an average of 12%.

Nutrition tips for a diet rich in magnesium

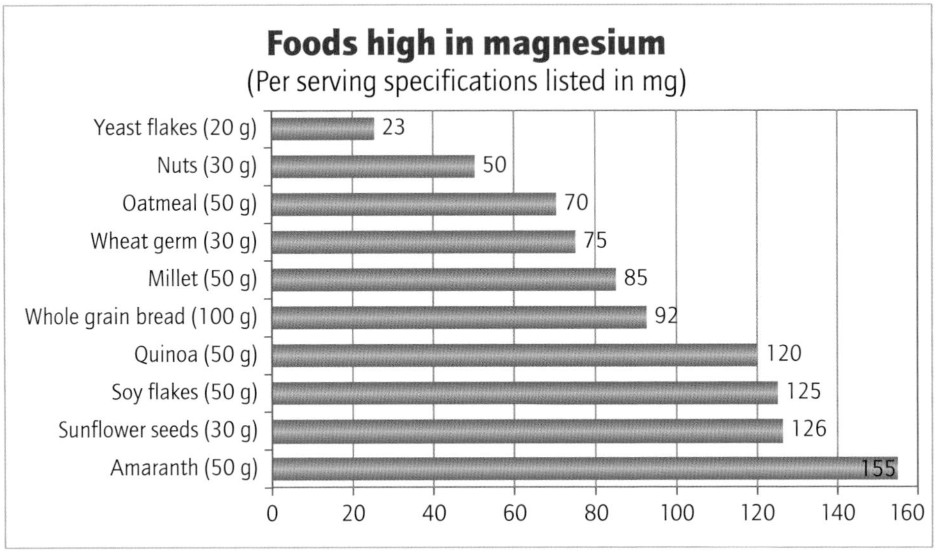

Foods high in magnesium
(Per serving specifications listed in mg)

Food	mg
Yeast flakes (20 g)	23
Nuts (30 g)	50
Oatmeal (50 g)	70
Wheat germ (30 g)	75
Millet (50 g)	85
Whole grain bread (100 g)	92
Quinoa (50 g)	120
Soy flakes (50 g)	125
Sunflower seeds (30 g)	126
Amaranth (50 g)	155

Fig. 63: Compiled from DGE nutrition panel, 43rd edition, 2005

- Mineral water with a magnesium content of more than 100 mg/l is recommended.

- A common mistake: taking magnesium right before a competition. This can be very hard on the gastrointestinal tract. We therefore always recommend regular doses after competing.

- Avoid taking magnesium during athletic exertion. Muscle cramps during athletic competitions are most often not caused by a magnesium deficiency but are the result of insufficient preparation and sodium deficiency due to over-exertion.

7.3 Iodine and selenium control thyroid function and thus the entire energy balance

Iodine and also selenium deficiencies can cause major thyroid problems in competitive athletes and are proven to cause extreme performance fluctuation and injuries.

Germany is known as an area of endemic iodine deficiency. The recommended supply of 200 µg of iodine via food, including iodized salt, lies at an average of 100 µg per day. The trace element iodine is a vital part of the thyroid hormones thyroxine (T_4) and Trijodthyronin (T_3), and thus is extremely important to the entire metabolism. With selenium as a co-factor the iodized thyroid hormone precursor trijodthyronin is converted to an active thyroid hormone (T_3).

Thyroid hormones are, among other things, extremely importantfor the division and growth of all cells, the carbohydrate, protein and fat metabolisms, the regulation of body temperature and the energy metabolism.

Any disruption of the thyroid hormone production affects the entire organism. An insufficient iodine supply causes a drop in the thyroid hormone level in the blood. The thyroid reacts with increased growth and enlarges. It tries to balance the lack of thyroid hormones by increasing production. A visible sign is the goiter at the neck, also called *struma*.

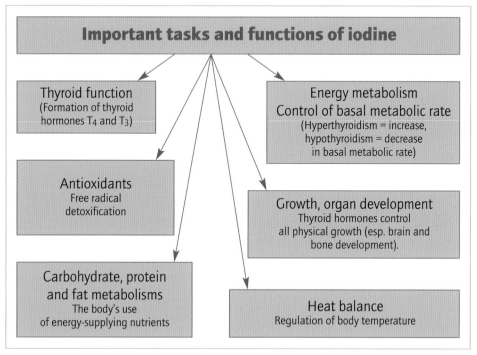

Fig. 64

Latent symptoms have been present in competitive athletes for along time – so far without clinical relevance

Athletes potentially have higher iodine requirements since they lose considerable amounts of iodine through perspiration. Testing of soccer players and high school students showed an iodine loss in sweat of up to 52 μg after playing for one hour (Mao et al, 2001).

According to our results, more than half the competitive athletes we examined had a latent hypofunction (hypothyroidism) of the thyroid. The athlete initially feels a little tired, cold sensitive and regularly experiences light night-sweats. After a period of time he feels listless and regenerates very slowly after intensive exertion. We frequently find these disorders even in young athletes. Iodine deficiency in athletic adolescents manifests itself in learning and concentration difficulties and frequent infections. Anyone with these symptoms should have his iodine supply checked.

Important information

Thyroid hormones are often significantly higher the day after major exertion due to intensive training and/or games. For this reason thyroid hormone tests are only expedient if no intensive athletic exertion occurred on the previous day.

Our tests

Blood test results of the 50 youth and junior national players from the unique European prevention program initiated by SALUTO/DHB, showed a 73% latent hypofunction with TSH-levels of > 4.3 μIU/ml. The players had reported frequent fatigue, night-sweats and poor regeneration ability for some time and described significant concentration difficulties throughout the day. Most players were still in school (some at a boarding school for athletes) and trained 10-18 hours per week.

An accurate interpretation of thyroid hormones in competitive athletes is extremely problematic. Thyroid hormone status can only be ascertained through blood tests. The TSH-level is an important indicator of thyroid hormone activity.

Our lab physicians assess a beginning latent hypothyroid condition (thyroid hypofunction) that does not yet require treatment, but can already cause malaise in competitive athletes (e.g. permanent fatigue, listlessness, night sweats, poor regeneration after intensive training or competition phases) at a TSH-level of > 2.8 µIU/ml. T_4 and T_3 were assessed in addition to the TSH-level.

In our experience TSH levels of > 2.8 µIU/ml can significantly impair the physical and mental performance in the long-term. After consulting our lab physicians we began by giving these competitive athletes 100-300 µg of Jodid separately (depending on thyroid hormone test results)in the morning, 20 minutes before breakfast. Subsequent thyroid hormone tests were done in regular intervals. In most of the competitive athletes thyroid hormone levels normalized with the specific use of varying doses of Jodid.

In some isolated cases the specific dose of Jodid did not suffice. After consulting with our lab physicians an appropriate medication was prescribed (e.g. thyroxin 50®). Regular thyroid hormone tests showed definite normalization.

In the future, SALUTO Institute and our partners will initiate additional research projects on competitive athletes with borderline thyroid hormone values and continue to critically examine our previous findings from a scientific standpoint.

Of the 9,150 competitive athletes only 15% showed a tendency to thyroid hyperfunction (hyperthyroidism). Our lab physicians assess a beginning latent hyperthyroidism that does not yet require treatment but can already cause malaise at a TSH-level of < 0.5 µIU/ml.

These athletes did not receive additional iodine in their customized micronutrient formulations.

The following illustration Fig 65 shows the difficulty in interpreting the initially measured TSH-level. According to our lab physicians a latent hypofunction exists at a TSH-level of > 2.5 µIU/ml. In our experience this can already represent preliminary performance-diminishing factors. Of crucial importance here is the monitoring of TSH-level trends over an extended period of time. These should also be compared to the athletes' subjective feeling of wellness.

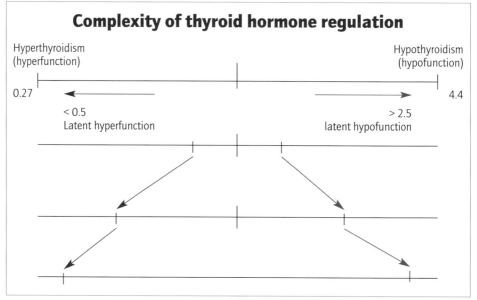

Fig. 65

The lab parameter iodine elimination

Another suitable lab parameter for measuring iodine status is iodine elimination in urine (urine iodine). Based on WHO criteria, the median urine iodine concentration in school-aged children and adults with an optimal iodine supply should be between 100-200 µg. For competitive athletes who train more than ten hours a day iodine intake can be much higher (up to 300 µg iodine).

A minor iodine deficiency (first degree) exists when iodine elimination lies between 50-99 µg/l. A moderate deficiency (second degree) exists in the area of 20-49 µg/l, and a major iodine deficiency (third degree) exists when less than < 20 µg/l iodine is eliminated with urine. For most competitive athletes supplementing between 100 to no more then 300 µg of iodine separately, depending on blood test results, is expedient.

Conclusions

Good thyroid hormone production (TSH-level < 2.5) ensures long-term optimal performance development in athletes. This absolutely must be taken into consideration for customized micronutrient formulations. Of the competitive athletes we examined 72% already showed signs of latent hypofunction that can be easily corrected with a specific supply of iodine (dosed according to thyroid hormone level). We recommend only taking iodine separately. For this reason micronutrient blends should not contain iodine.

In our experience a TSH-level > 2.8 µIU/ml can lead to long-term adverse effects on physical and mental performance.

However, when thyroid hormones and also cellular selenium concentrations are at optimal levels the following thyroid functions can become apparent:

• stimulation of cell division and differentiation,

• boosting of anabolic metabolism status with positive nitrogen balance,

• regulation of energy conversion in carbohydrate and fat metabolism,

• activation of protein biosynthesis in liver, muscles, brain and other organs and

• hormonal safeguarding of basal metabolic rate.

A case study

As an example, the author's long-standing, latent hypothyroidism (hypofunction): Every day around 5:30 am, I begin my day with strength training followed by 45 to 50 minutes of endurance training.

At age 47, I suddenly noticed a drastic increase in fatigue and listlessness. I began to have night sweats. In addition I quickly began to feel constricted in the elevator and felt increasingly depressed. I immediately had my thyroid hormone level checked. According to the lab physicians I had an acceptable

---

level of 3.3 µIU/ml. I showed this to an internist friend and asked for his help. He explained that at my age initial hormonal changes take place that may be typical andropausal ailments. The basal TSH-level combined with T_3 and T_4 were at acceptable levels.

During the many years I worked with athletes I often heard these same complaints. I therefore decided to practice exactly what I had been doing successfully with athletes. Every morning I took 3 x 100 µg of Jodid ten minutes before breakfast. After three weeks all of my symptoms had disappeared and after six weeks the basal TSH-level had normalized at 1.8 µIU/ml.

Selenium

Next to iodine selenium is essential to the thyroid hormone synthesis. An iodine deficiency in the thyroid causes increased formation of toxic hydroperoxides that are rendered harmless by selenium-containing glutathione peroxidase. Thyroid

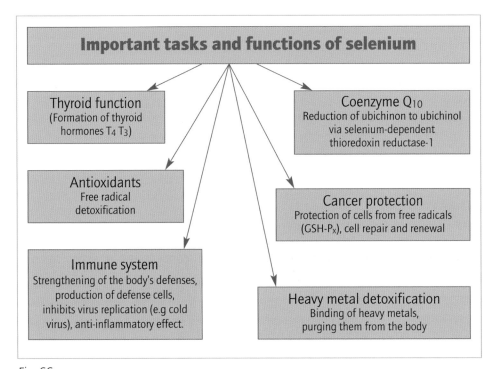

Fig. 66

dysfunction can also be caused by a selenium deficiency. The active thyroid hormone trijodthyronin (T$_3$) cannot be formed without selenium. Thus thyroid hypofunction can be caused not only by an iodine deficiency, but also a selenium deficiency.

Selenium occurs in all of the body's cells and fluids. It is most concentrated in the thyroid, kidneys, liver, spleen, heart and prostate. Selenium is a functional component of many enzymes and proteins (selenium protein). The key enzyme of the body's natural defenses against freeradicals, glutathione peroxidase, is selenium-dependent. Glutathione peroxidase renders toxic peroxides harmless with the aid of selenium and prevents damage to the genetic material of the cells (DNA) by free radicals. The high susceptibility to infection in competitive athletes is in part due to very low cellular selenium concentrations. Selenium can repair cell damage via repair enzymes.

Selenium deficiency is very common in Germany

Germany and many other countries rank among the selenium-poor areas of Europe. Even with a balanced diet an adult gets barely more than 45 µg of selenium per day because our foods generally contain little selenium. Seafood, giblets, green tea and Brazil nuts are good sources of selenium.

We found blatant cellular deficiencies in the competitive athletes we examined. A good selenium status has a positive effect on immune system stability, regeneration ability and capacity. A good selenium status requires a daily dose of approximately 1.5-2 µg of selenium per kg of body weight. A sensible dose always depends on the individual cellular selenium status. Long-term use of more then 200 µg can cause toxic reactions.

Dosage recommendations for selenium

Ascertainment of intracellular selenium concentration (in erythrocytes) is absolutely necessary because the serum concentration is almost always in the normal range, while intraerythrocytic selenium concentrations show definite deficiencies (see pg. 39). Intracellular selenium concentrations should not exceed 190 µg/Ery.

Organic selenium preparations (selenium yeast, selenomethionine) of up to 200 µg are particularly suitable for endurance athletes as a nutritional supplement. A long-term higher dosage > 200 µg should be avoided due to previously mentioned possible toxic reactions. But inorganic selenium preparations (sodium selenite, sodium selenate) can also be used as supplements and for therapy in cases of selenium deficiencies. (Note: take on empty stomach, take sodium selenite more than one hour before or after vitamin C).

7.4   Potassium

Potassium is one of the body's most important intracellular minerals. Most of the potassium, 60%, is contained in the muscle cells. The potassium balance depends on adequate magnesium. Potassium is transported to the cells with the aid of magnesium-dependent enzymes Na+/K ± ATPase. Magnesium deficiency causes the cells to lose potassium.

Potassium is critical to:

*   energy metabolism (energy production and storage (ATP), cellular absorption of glucose and formation of muscle glycogen)

*   monitoring acid-base balance and volume of cellular fluid,

*   maintainingelasticity of vascular and skeletal musculature, muscle cell contraction and stimulation,

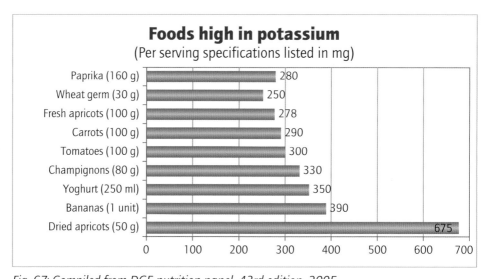

Foods high in potassium
(Per serving specifications listed in mg)

Food	mg
Paprika (160 g)	280
Wheat germ (30 g)	250
Fresh apricots (100 g)	278
Carrots (100 g)	290
Tomatoes (100 g)	300
Champignons (80 g)	330
Yoghurt (250 ml)	350
Bananas (1 unit)	390
Dried apricots (50 g)	675

Fig. 67: Compiled from DGE nutrition panel, 43rd edition, 2005

- the cells (activation of cells, stabilization of cell membranes),

- the nerve cells (regulation of excitatory impulses and transmission of nerve impulses) and for

- the enzymes (activation of different enzymes).

A diet high in potassium and magnesium forms the basis for a smooth metabolic process. Daily consumption of potassium should be between 2,000-3,000 mg from fruit and vegetables.

Athletes need more potassium

Athletes have high potassium requirements because they lose an appreciable amount of potassium (approx. 300 mg per liter) with sweat. During physical exertion potassium ions shift from intracellular to extracellular, meaning the potassium concentration in the blood rises. In addition an abundant amount of potassium is released into the muscles during breakdown of glycogen.

Potassium is needed particularly for glycogen storage during the regeneration phase. Potassium is stored in the musculature together with glycogen (approx. 19.5 mg of potassium per g of glycogen). The potassium component in sports drinks should be approx. 100-250 mg per liter of beverage. Not too much potassium (300 mg/l sports drink) should be replenished during the exertion phase because, as previously mentioned, the potassium level in the blood rises. A potassium level that is too high has a negative effect on physical capacity and increases the risk of arrhythmia.

When perspiring heavily during extremely high temperatures it is advisable to drink a glass of water with one half of a *Kalinor®* effervescent tablet (available at pharmacies) dissolved in it. This facilitates rapid replenishment of glycogen stores in the liver and musculature.

7.5   Chromium

Chromium is a co-factor in the insulin response and as such participates in the regulation of blood sugar level (glucose tolerance), glycogen synthesis and the absorption of amino acids into the muscle tissue.

Chromium's function is:

- boosting glycogen formation in liver and musculature,

- conservation of glycogen during exertion,

- regulation of blood sugar level,

- optimization of fat metabolism, and

- facilitates weight loss

Increased chromium deficiencies in athletes

Intensive physical exertion causes increased chromium elimination in urine and chromium loss in sweat. Increased chromium loss in urine through sports is twice to five times as high as that of non-athletes. In our experience chromium deficiencies can often be found in competitive athletes. A full blood count of < 98 mmol/l can verifiably delay glycogen formation in the liver and musculature.

Dosage recommendations for chromium

Recommended dosage for competitive athletes is between 100 to 400 µg of chromium. Since carbohydrates are the most important energy source for any intensive endurance performance, a sufficient chromium supply is essential for

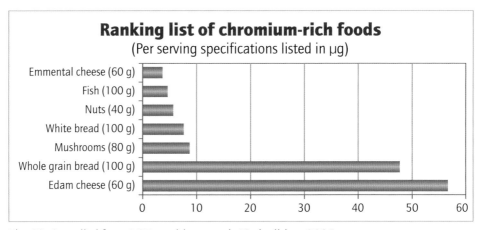

Fig. 68: Compiled from DGE nutrition panel, 43rd edition, 2005

tapping into one's possible potential. An insufficient chromium supply means a low glycogen reserve level and thus a low power reserve. In contrast, it is our experience that a sufficient chromium supply can clearly improve glycogen storage. A sufficient chromium supply ensures the glycogen supply and thus conserves glycogen stores, which can be a crucial advantage during exertion that lasts for several hours. Endurance athletes should therefore eat a diet especially high in chromium. Foods high in chromium are whole grain products, nuts, Edam and Emmentaler cheese (see Fig. 68).

7.6   Vitamin C

Endurance athletes have considerably higher vitamin C requirements. Vitamin C also has a stabilizing effect in the maintenance of various connective tissue functions. Vitamin C is a powerful antioxidant that protects vital cell building blocks and organs from oxidative damage through free radicals. The antioxidative functions of vitamin C closely interact on abiochemical level with those of coenzyme (Q_{10}), vitamin E, gluthathione and selenium.

Tasks and functions of vitamin C:

* immune system: activity and power of defense cells.

* antioxidant: water-soluble antioxidant, protects cell membranes, organs, protein and other vitamins from free radicals.

* collagen production: formation and stabilization of connective tissue (muscles, bones, blood vessels, etc.)

* controls histamine levels: histamine plays a key role in allergies (e.g. hay fever)

* neurotransmitters (nerve messenger substance): production of neurotransmitters important to restful sleep and psychological equilibrium (serotonin).

* iron utilization: improves absorption and utilization.

* folic acid: activation into metabolic form.

Important protective function for athletes

In the past few years we have continuously seen a functional link between the effects of a targeted vitamin C supply and a verifiable decrease in injury risk. When competitive athletes had a blood vitamin-C-level level between 150 and 200 µmol/l the injury risk could be decreased considerably.

Especially the increase of pyridinium in athletes engaging in intensive physical exertion without a specific micronutrient formulation and the increased formation of free radicals, show initial degenerative changes in many connective tissue structures (ligaments, tendon and ligament apparatus) (see pg. 107-109). Therefore a sufficient vitamin C supply makes particular sense, even if this continues to be a subject of great controversy.

Dosage recommendations for vitamin C

We gave competitive athletes between 500 and 3,000 mg orally in the form of customized micronutrient formulations. The amountof vitamin C given depends on the results of a blood test.

Vitamin C infusions are a good choice for boosting regeneration during the early stages of an infection, but of course only after consulting the attending physician. The advantages of infusions over oral vitamin C doses are the vigorous activation of immune cells (e.g. phagocytes) and the avoidance of gastrointestinal problems. During phases of particularlyintense competition competitive athletes with a verifiably high susceptibility to infection are given regularly scheduled treatments with vitamin C infusions (e.g. 7.5-15 g of vitamin C in 100-200 ml = 0.9% NaCl, two to three times per week over a two-week period) based on the doctor's special recommendation, to optimize the immune system.

7.7 Omega-3 fatty acids

The most important omega-3 fatty acids include alpha-linolenic acid, eicosapentaenoic acid (EPA) and docosahexaenoic acid (DHA). Alpha-linolenic acid, the "parent" fatty acid in the omega-3 fatty acid metabolism, can be found in ferns, mosses and some plant-based oils such as linseed and rapeseed oil. The human organism can barely transform the short-chain alpha-linolenic acid (approx. 5-10%) into EPA and DHA. For this reason the health-promoting effects of EPA and DHA cannot be attained by taking plant-based alpha-linolenic acid.

EPA and DHA are indispensible components of each cell membrane and thus are largely responsible for good health: they:

- strengthen the immune system,

- have an anti-inflammatory effect,

- support oxygen supply to organs,

- lower elevated blood lipids, and

- improve concentration and mental capacity.

Our body produces insufficient amounts of these two essential fatty acids in our metabolism. For this reason we must get a regular sufficient supply from the food we consume. Unfortunately the excessive consumption of omega-6 fatty acids in our foods and the much too low omega-3 fatty acid content have been known for some time. The ratio of omega-6 to omega-3 fatty acids in the Eskimo's food supply is 1:1, while that of Europeans is approximately 20-50:1.

Competitive athletes
often have an omega-3 deficiency

Due to omega-3 fatty acid's (EPA, DHA) many important tasks their significance is still being underestimated in competitive sports today.

The significance of omega-3 fatty acids in metabolic functions can be described as follows:

- immune system (strengthens immune defense, modulates inflammation metabolism (anti-inflammatory effect),

- neurotransmitters (regulates the neurotransmitter metabolism in the brain, mental stability and strength),

- energy metabolism (improves blood flow characteristics, decreases blood viscosity and risk of thrombosis) and

- heart muscle (increases heart muscle capacity, anti-arrhythmic effect).

For optimal diagnostics of omega-3 fatty acids the erythrocyte membrane lipids should be measured on an empty stomach, because fatty acid distribution is subject to considerable nutrition-related fluctuations. Ordinarily this measurement/material is done with plasma from a fasting patient/gc. The normal range in plasma is: alpha-linolenic acid 15-30 mg/l, EPA 20-55 mg/l, DHA 50-110 mg/l.

Background information

Interesting new developments unrelated to competitive sports: A so-called *omega-3 index* has been created that represents a new risk factor for cardiovascular complications all the way to cardiac death. According to long-term studies, if the percentage of these two omega-3 fatty acids (EPA, DHA) in the erythrocytes is < 4%, the risk of sudden cardiac death is 10 x higher than it is with an omega-3 index of > 8%. The next few years will show how the interpretation of this omega-3 index will continue to evolve and to what extent these results will be acceptably supported from a scientific standpoint.

Dosage recommendations for omega-3 fatty acids

When taking omega-3 fatty acids (EPA, DHA) it is important to also have a good supply of vitamin E, selenium and coencyme Q_{10}. Competitive athletes should take 1,000 to 2,000 mg of omega-3 fatty acids.

The quality of omega-3 fatty acids is of basic significance. The purity of products is particularly important. Many apparently reasonable omega-3 fatty acids advertised as high-quality products stem from fish that are raised in small areas at large breeding facilities and are given antibiotics and in some instances growth hormones. To create omega-3 fatty acids of truly optimal quality the oil should come from offshore fish in large bodies of water. There are very few pure products that meet these criteria. To our competitive athletes we therefore recommend EPA concentrations of at least 420 mg and DHA concentrations of 280 mg. The recommended dosage is 1-2 capsules daily, depending on training intensity and blood test results.

The following foods contain omega-3 fatty acids:

Table 7: Omega-3 fatty acid content per 100 g

Linolenic acid	
Linseed oil	54.2 g
Rapeseed oil	9.2 g
Eicosapentaenoic acid	
Herring	2.3 g
Salmon	0.65 g
Mackerel	0.95 g

Compiled from DGE nutrition panel, 43rd edition, 2005

7.8 L-carnitine

L-carnitine is a natural substance. The human body stores approximately 20-25 g of L-carnitine, particularly in skeletal muscles and the heart. L-carnitine occurs primarily in meat and stems from the Latin word carnis (flesh). Plant-derived foods contain very little carnitine. A balanced, non-vegetarian diet such as the western mixed diet supplies us with about 100-300 mg of L-carnitine per day. However, over the last ten years L-carnitine consumption from food has decreased by about 20% in Europe and the United States. This is largely due to a decrease in beef consumption.

L-carnitine's function in the body

At this time there are numerous scientific studies on the various positive effects of a targeted L-carnitine supply. Scientists describe improved muscular regeneration after athletic exertion and certain immunomodulating effects with regular use of L-carnitine in sports with doses of 1,000 to 2,000 mg (Billigman, Siebrecht 2004).

L-carnitine plays a central part in the transport and burning of long-chain fatty acids. Energy production from fats, the so-called *fat burning*, takes place in the cell powerhouses, the mitochondria. When energy is going to be produced from fat the fatty acids first have to reach the mitochondria, and they cannot do so without help. L-carnitine sees to it that fatty acids are transported to the mitochondria.

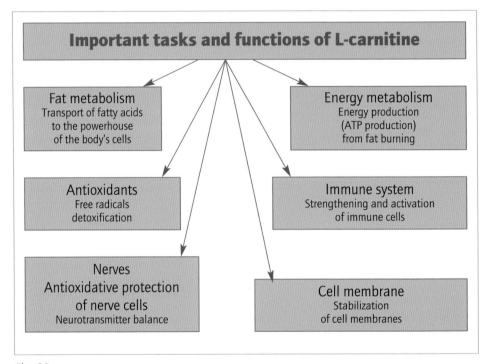

Fig. 69

In fact, two independent research groups were able to prove in two different studies that taking *Carnipure*™ as a nutritional supplement stimulates long-chain fatty acid metabolism in healthy adults (Müller et al, 2002; Wutzke et al 2004). The test subjects received marked fatty acids with a meal before as well as after adding *Carnipure*™ nutritional supplement for 10-days. Afterwards marked CO_2 was measured in the exhalation air as a degradation product of the marked fatty acids. The scientists observed a significant increase of marked CO_2 in the exhalation air, indicating a definite increase of fat burning in healthy adults after using *Carnipure*™.

Through its central role in the metabolism L-carnitine takes on a series of protective functions against metabolic disruptions on the cellular level. Next to mitochondrial transport and oxidative breakdown of fatty aicds, the detoxification of mitochondria from toxic metabolic products and the protection of the mitochondrial membrane play a major role. In addition L-carnitine possesses distinct antioxidative characteristics.

All energy carriers, meaning carbohydrates, fats and proteins, are activated in our metabolism with the bond to coenzyme A. L-carnitine regulates the availability of coenzyme A, thereby supporting the glucose and amino acid metabolism.

L-carnitine for active athletes

Many scientific tests show the positive effects of *Carnipure*™ in professional athletes and active individuals. Performance is optimized, fatigue symptoms are delayed and the regeneration process is accelerated. L-carnitine decreases amino acid breakdown and promotes the forming of lean muscle mass. L-carnitine is like an internal training program. It sustains the enjoyment of athletic activity and eases the transition to an exertion phase.

Scientists were able to show through different studies that Carnipure™ tartrate as a nutritional supplement has a positive effect on regeneration after athletic exertion on young as well as older test subjects (Spiering et al, 2007 and 2008; Ho et al, 2010; Volek et al, 2002; Kraemer et al, 2005). Different parameters that are typically elevated after athletic exertion were not as high, or rather returned to normal levels more quickly. In addition muscle soreness was definitely reduced. This positive effect became more pronounced with an increased daily dose, but was already obvious with a daily dose of 1 g L-carnitine. "*Carnipure*™ can play a major role in the nutrition of athletes and have a positive effect on their health", says William Kraemer, author of this study.

Indispensible to the immune system

The cells in our immune system depend on the availability of L-carnitine, on the one hand for their own energy supply of fatty acids, and on the other hand for constant modulation of their membrane structures into which fatty acids and other membrane building blocks must be permanently embedded. An increased immune activity after intensive athletic exertionleads to reparable inflammatory reactions and to a significant drop of L-carnitine in the blood since much more L-carnitine is being eliminated via the kidneys.

Insufficient metabolic availability of L-carnitnie (L-carnitine sufficiency) interferes with the cellular energy (ATP) supply from fat burning, inhibits coenzyme-A-dependent metabolic processes, increases the risk of mitochondrial damage, and weakens the immune system.

Assessing the L-carnitine status

The ratio of esterified acyl-carnitine (AC) to free L-carnitine (FC) is a parameter that provides a good description of the L-carnitine status and indicates an L-carnitine insufficiency, or rather the insufficient availability of free L-carnitine. An AC/FC quotient in the blood of < 0.4 is considered normal. If the AC/FC ratio increases to > 0.4 it is considered a L-carnitine insufficiency. Major and intensive athletic exertion such as in competitive sports causes increased formation of acyl-carnitines in blood and tissues. For this reason the ratio of acyl-carnitine (AC) to free L-carnitine (AC/FC) increases. Since the kidneys reabsorb acyl-carnitine (AC) less well than free L-carnitine, there is a higher carnitine loss via the urine. A level of 40-75 µmol/l I considered a good plasma L-carnitine supply.

Dosage recommendations for L-carnitine

Important information: Many endurance athletes frequently have a low ferritin level along with a simultaneous low L-carnitine status in the blood and musculature. A suboptimal iron status manifests itself through the same symptoms (e.g. quick onset of fatigue, decreased endurance capacity) as insufficient L-carnitine availability. We recommend regular blood tests to assess the AC/FC ratio.

When we tested competitive athletes with a balanced diet we also measured AC/FC quotients of > 6. These indicate an existing carnitine insufficiency. A targeted supplement can correct this sufficiency. The quality of the L-carnitine is of particular importance. We recommend products containing Carnipure™ as a raw material (www.carnipure-for-you.com).

7.9 Creatine – we will forgo additional supply

At this point we will deliberately forgo a detailed scientific examination of creatine's significance in the performance development of athletes. More than 100 different studies are already in existence.

A description of the significance of the creatine metabolism in the area of energy production can be found on the following pages. There is no micronutrient that is subject to more controversy than creatine. There are a number of select studies on increasing athletic performance through creatine. According to international scientists and the board of the Anti-Doping Commission, creatine will soon be put on the list of banned substances. Athletes from many different sports currently use creatine regularly in varying doses.

AM-formula blend boosts
the creatine phosphate metabolism

It is our experience that an optimal customized micronutrient formulation containing high-quality amino acids (AM-formula blend) considerably enhances the replenishment of creatine phosphatestores.

A specific supply of this AM-formula blend based on the athlete's individual requirements of between 30 and 70 g would not only be enough to optimize the creatine phosphate metabolism, but also to verifiably stabilize the many connective tissue structures (ligaments, tendons, cartilage). The following illustration shows, among other things, how the amino acids arginine, methionine, etc., support the synthesis and formation of creatine phosphate.

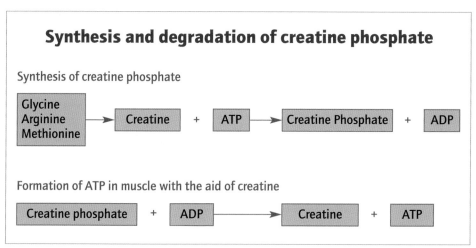

Fig. 70

7.10 Content and significance of other micronutrients in a customized micronutrient formulation

Zeaxanthin

Zeaxanthin together with lutein is one of the most important protective agents for the preservation of vision in old age and for competitive athletes. Particularly important are the so-called oxycarotenoidsthat protect the macula lutea, the yellow spot in the central retina, from oxidation and thus from macular degeneration (AMD).

PABA

Para-aminobenzoic acid, or PABA, is a natural water-soluble cofactor of the B-group vitamins. The antioxidants protect the body from solar radiation. PABA keeps the skin smooth and supple and accelerates the healing of burn wounds.

Inositol

Inositol, like choline, is involved in the formation of the cell membrane. Beyond that this substance serves as a signal substance in the transmission of commands to the cell. It benefits the health and growth of hair. A propensity to eczema is often due to an inositol deficiency.

Silicium

Silicium is an ultratrace element, and indispensible for cross-linking of protein and mucopolysaccharides, which are swellable structural substances for fiber-forming agents in the body. This mineral is an important nutrient for bones, cartilage, connective tissue, hair and nails. The presence of silicium affects the mineralization process of the bone. Silicium shares responsibility for the elasticity and stability of the arterial walls, increases lung volume and has an anti-inflammatory effect.

Choline

This substance is a phospholipid component, and as such provides structure to all cell membranes. In the brain and nerves choline is transformed into acetylcholine, the important neurotransmitter in stimulus transmission. As a necessary component of gallbladder secretion, choline emulsifies the nutritional fats and participates in the elimination of triglycerides (fats) from the liver. In addition choline boosts the liver's detoxification capacity. Choline enhances memory function.

Bioflavonoids, citrus flavonoids

Flavonoids affect the organism in many different ways. They have a positive effect on the circulation and memory function, they protect healthy tissue from radiation, have some ability to inhibit bacteria or stop viral growth,and lower the histamine level. Histamine is a tissue hormone that is involved in many regulatory processes. When athletes with allergies are exposed to "their" allergen their histamine level goes up dramatically. Flavonoids also reduce the lactate level in the muscles and improve the iodine supply. The have an anti-inflammatory effect and lower the body temperature. Flavonoids increase the effectiveness and bioavailability of vitamin C.

Green tea extract

Green tea contains a series of polyphenol bonds that display a strong antioxidative affect. The most wellknown among these is epigallocatechingallat (EGCG), which has a positive effect on the cardiovascular system. Green tea relieves the body's own antioxidative system.

Red wine extract/OPC

Red wine extract is an especially effective blend of antioxidative bioflavonoids with red wine's ability to protect blood vessels. The strong antioxidative capacity of the oligomeric proanthocyanidins (OPC) it contains is far superior to that of vitamin C and vitamin E, and has an anti-inflammatory effect.

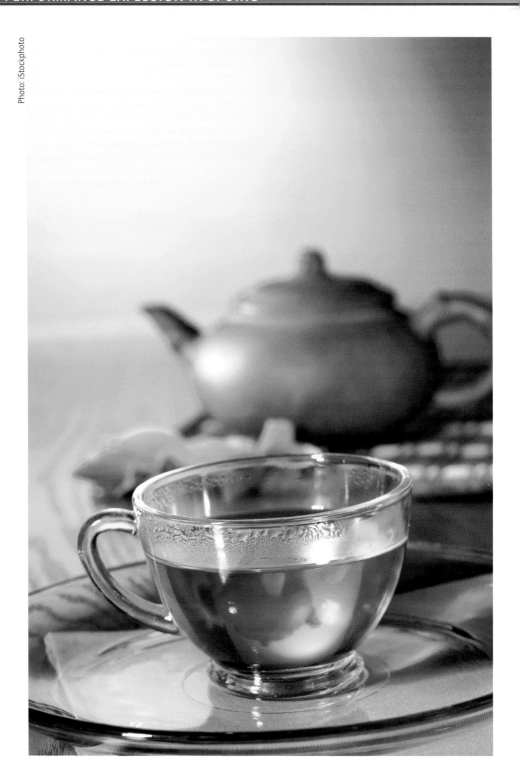

Dietary fiber

Guar

Guar is the base for the granular customized HCK® micronutrient blend. As a cold water-soluble, purely plant-based and highly swellable fiber, guar flour is the "cellular key" to micronutrients. Guar flour is made from the seeds of the Indian cluster bean plant. The highly purified pharmaceutical-quality flour forms a natural matrix in which micronutrients can be embedded. After the micronutrient blend is ingested with a liquid the granulate swells in the gastrointestinal tract and forms a large gel-like surface, a "colloidal system". The nutrients embedded there can be accessed for hours. Guar flour itself serves the body as indigestible fiber with proven benefits to the intestinal flora.

HPM-cellulose

Together with hemicellulose, pectin and lignin form cellulose, the main component in plant-based dietary fiber.

Inulin

Inulin serves as food for the natural intestinal bacteria. Regular use results in an improved intestinal flora.

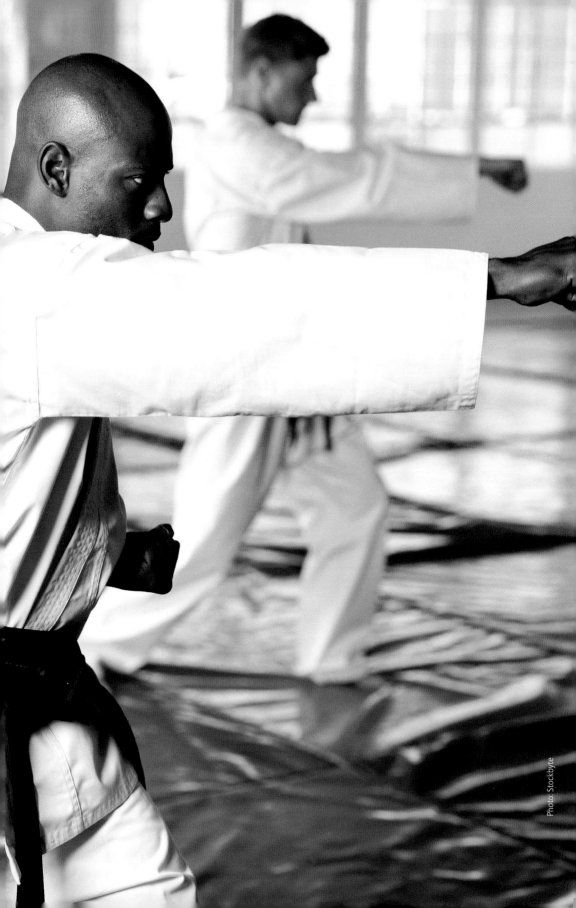

8   The anti-doping concept in practice

8.1   Brief characterization of the customized micronutrient formulation

Definition

These micronutrient formulations serve the functional maintenance (including mental and physical capacity) of many physiological metabolic functions and the stabilization of connective tissue structures (ligaments, tendons, cartilage structures). The highest priority is a balanced diet as defined by DGE.

Active substances and active substance groups

These are physiological micronutrients that naturally occur in the body (e.g. iron, L-carnitine, and more) and their active substance groups (vitamins, vitaminoids, minerals trace elements, essential fatty acids and amino acids).

Purpose of customized micronutrient formulations

- compensation of growing micronutrient losses (necessary due to the proven greenhouse effect, in spite of a balanced diet),

- performance optimization and performance continuity through training without injury,

- performance increase through proven decrease in injuries without external force;

- long-term stabilization of many stressed connective tissue structures (ligaments, tendons and cartilage structures),

- optimization of energy metabolism because increasing detection of micronutrient deficiencies in competitive athletes can lead to growing metabolizing of the body's own protein structures;

- optimization of physiological metabolism resulting in better health and thus guaranteed training continuity;

- stabilization of immune system, definite reduction in missed training sessions/competitions due to infection;

- improved mental and physical capacity;

- competitive sports has an important role model function for young people. The anti-doping concept presents options for achieving top performances in all sports without major injuries;

- considerably improved image of competitive/elite sports with the aid of the anti-doping concept.

Mode of action

Micronutrients verifiably optimize natural metabolic processes and are able to stabilize many connective tissue structures.

Side effects

There are no physiological side effects in the represented dosage (see pg. 246ff.). Minor skin irritation can occur in cases of existing skin allergies (psoriasis,

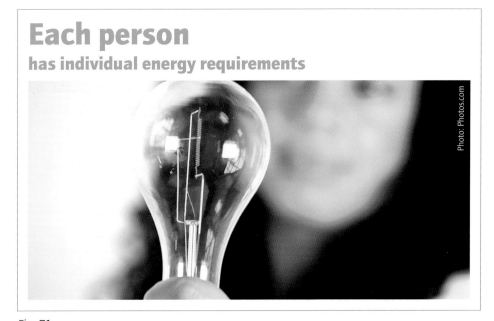

Each person

has individual energy requirements

Photo: Photos.com

Fig. 71

neurodermatitis); important exceptions to be considered (e.g. vitamin A, vitamin D, selenium).

8.2 General criteria for the use of micronutrient

A balanced diet is a basic requirement for competitive sports. It also guarantees a good base-acid ratio, which is critical to the athletes' absorption of micronutrients. Additional details about the three-day base-acid profile can be found on pg. 226.

Important information

Intensive training and competition phases can cause microbleeding in the gastrointestinal tract, preventing maximal micronutrient absorption. If an athlete complains of increasing fatigue, additional intravenous electrolyte infusions can be wise. However, this should be discussed with the attending physician on an individual basis.

Customized micronutrient formulation

Individually prepared micronutrient formulation – contingent on results of

- Intracellular and other blood tests – the existing database with results from 9,150 top and 6, 434 recreational athletes,

- The percent deviation from the respective median value of the micronutrient concentrations (the many connective tissue structures stabilize at > 20% above the respective median value),

- The nutrition analysis,

- The specially developed protocol sheet for the competitive athlete,

- Type of sport and training content (ratio of endurance/strength/coordination/flexibility),

- Differentiation in training and competition phases,

- Age structure and

- Absorption ability of the gastrointestinal tract

Fig. 72

Table 8: Reference ranges for micronutrient concentrations in customized micronutrient formulations

Customized micronutrient formulation (See criteria on pg. 171, fig. 72)			
Active ingredient per day	**Daily dose**	**Active ingredient**	**Daily dose**
Vitamins		**Trace elements**	
Vitamin A (retinol)	0.8-1.5 mg (1,000-3,600 i.u.)	Chromium	100-250 µg
		Manganese	5-20 mg
Vitamin B$_1$ (thiamine)	10-70 mg	Molybdenum	50-200 µg
Vitamin B$_2$ (riboflavin)	10-70 mg	Selenium	50-200 µg
Vitamin B$_6$ (pyridoxine)	20-80 mg	Zinc	12-48 mg
Vit. B$_{12}$ (cyanocobalamine)	30-400 µg	**Minerals**	
Vitamin C (ascorbic acid)	0.2 g-2 g	Calcium	200-800 mg
Vitamin D$_3$	5-20 µg	Potassium	200-400 mg
Natural Vitamin E	150-400 mg	Magnesium	200-600 mg
From alpha tocopherol	85-340 mg	Silicium	20-60 mg
Gamma tocoperhol	13-53 mg	**Quasi vitamins**	
Natural carotinoids	8 mg	Choline	80-240 mg
From alpha carotene	70 µg	Coenzyme Q$_{10}$	30-100 mg
		Inositol	60-180 mg
Beta carotene	1.9 mg	L-carnitine	250-1,000 mg
Cryptoxanthine	15 µg	PABA	20-80 mg
Leutin	6.0 mg	**Plant extracts**	
Zeaxanthin	15.0 µg	Green tea extract	350.8 mg
Biotin (vitamin H)	45-150.0 µg	Citrus bioflavinoids	375.9 mg
Folic acid (vitamin B$_9$)	0.4-1.6 mg	Red wine extract	350.8 mg
Niacin (Vitamin B$_3$)	10-60 mg	**Fiber**	
Pantothenic acid	20-80 mg	Guar flour	3,585.7 mg
With iodine*	50-200 µg	HPM cellulose	139.6 mg
Daily intake mode: Example: 3 scoops: 1.5 scoops morning and afternoon		Inulin	184.2 mg
		Additional amino acids in special cases Arginine	1,000-3,000 mg
		Glutamine	500-3,000 mg

* In case of borderline TSH-level (T$_3$, T$_4$) towards hypofunction and existing symptoms, an isolated dose of iodide 10 minutes before breakfast is recommended (dosage based on thyroid blood test).

Dosage and intake mode of AM-formula blend

In addition to customized micronutrient formulations the competitive athletes receive varying doses of the high-quality AM-formula blend (based on blood test results).

Daily doses are between 30-70 g for the stabilization of many connective tissue structures (ligaments, tendons, various cartilage structures).

Table 9: Doses of 30-70 g of high-quality amino acid blend (AM-formula blend)

Amino acids	Specifications for the intake of 30-70 g (AM-formula blend)
L-alanine	2.4-5.6
L-arginine	2.8-6.9
L-aspartic acid	1.7-4.0
L-glutamic acid	4.1-9.5
L-glycine	6.0-14.0
L-histidine	0.4-0.92
L-isoleucine	1.40-3.3
L-leucine	1.8-4.2
L-lysine	1.1-2.5
L-methionine	0.2-0.4
L-phenylalanine	0.6-1.4
L-proline	3.84-9.0
L-serin	0.5-1.2
L-threonine	0.5-1.3
L-tyrosine	0.3-0.70
L-valine	1.9-4.4

In our experience the intake mode should be as follows: in the morning with breakfast, directly after each training session, in the evening two hours before bedtime (one generous Tbs equals approx. 10 g). This amino acid blend should be stirred into an electrolyte beverage and consumed directly after training.

Additional micronutrients

Tryptophan

The amino acid blend intentionally contains no tryptophan since it is proven to cause increased fatigue. Our research results show blatant tryptophan deficiencies in competitive athletes. We therefore recommended that the athletes take 1-2 x 500 mg in the evening, two hours before bedtime, after intensive training and competition phases. The athletes confirmed that both their sleep and general mood had improved. Long-term deficiencies in the amino acid L-tryptophan can significantly decrease quality of sleep and thereby delay the important regeneration phase.

Omega-3 fatty acids

Depending on workload and blood count, we gave the competitive athletes an additional 1,000 to 2,000 mg omega-3 fatty acids. These have a proven anti-inflammatory effect and can thus stabilize the immune system.

Iron

A specific iron supply (e.g. well-tolerated *ferro sanol duodenal*®, etc.) was given every day after dinner for 3-4 weeks. After that time the athletes took iron only 2-3 times a week until the next blood test (after 6-8 weeks). Long-term medication with iron is counterproductive to the stabilization of the immune system.

Iodine

After consulting with physicians, isolated doses of iodine were given in cases of proven borderline TSH-levels towards hypofunction of the thyroid with respective symptoms present, until the nextcheck-up. The iodine dose was taken in the morning, 10 minutes before breakfast.

60% of examined athletes had a tendency toward thyroid hypofunction with accompanying symptoms such as fatigue, night sweats and a certain amount of listlessness. In some cases even a targeted iodine supply was no longer sufficient to normalize thyroid hormones.Consultation with advising physicians necessarily resulted in appropriate medication.

Magnesium

In addition we gave the athletes a specific supply of magnesium in the form of orotate (*magnerot classic®*) chewable tablets in doses of 9 x 35 mg a day, depending on intracellular blood test results.

Important information: if the athlete takes iron with food in the evening, a reasonable dose of magnesium two hours later would be recommended.

Glucosamine sulfate and chondroitin sulfate

During intensive preparation and competition phases the competitive athletes also take the joint-building micronutrients glucosamine sulfate and chondroitin sulfate for prevention purposes, isolated as a combination preparation (see pg. 72-73).

Table 10: Dosage recommendation

Micronutrient	Prevention
Glucosamine sulfate	1,500 (e.g. 2 x 750 mg/day) as interval therapy during high exertion phases (e.g. competition preparation)
Chondroitin sulfate	400-1,200 mg (e.g. 2 x 400 mg/day) as interval therapy during high exertion phases (e.g. competition preparation)

8.3 Important details about the use of micronutrients in competitive sports

Experts

Only experts (physicians with emphasis on sports medicine, sport scientists, nutritionists and pharmacists) should undertake targeted supplementation with micronutrients. An optimal combination of individual micronutrient concentrations is only possible through intracellular blood tests. These are very complex and expensive and are therefore rarely done. However, next to the special cellular blood test an appropriately large database with the results of competitive athletes is recommend, which also facilitates an adequate assessment of the blood tests (see pg. 180). Various other aspects of micronutrient supplementation can be found in the chapter "Fairytales and myths" (see pg. 15-20).

Proven benefits

The metabolic benefits of respective preparations should be scientifically traceable. Previous dosage recommendations by DGE and the German Society for Sports Medicine and Prevention (DGSP) are rather dismissive with respect to dietary supplements and have no verifiable effect on lowering the high injury risk of competitive athletes (see pg. 100-102).

Dosage recommendations

The previously recommended supply is purely based on fundamental considerations regarding the relationship between energy use and increased nutrient requirements. The specified recommendations are joint recommendations by German-speaking nutrition societies (Germany, Austria, Switzerland). To date there is a considerable lack of sports medical exercise-physiological data for the practical review of the clinical relevance of previous dosage recommendations.

Injury risk – optimizing performance

The loss of nutrients in plants due to the described greenhouse effect (see pg. 40-43) and the increased metabolizing of the body's own protein structures for the athlete's energy production (see pg. 82-85), makes a targeted supply of micronutrients urgently necessary in order to minimize the high injury risk in competitive athletes and to thereby achieve long-term performance consistency.

Individuality

Every athlete has his personal micronutrient requirements. This should be measured with the described valid intracellular lab and diagnostics tests and other blood analyses (see pg. 171, Fig 72). An individually adapted, targeted micronutrient supply makes sense.

Balanced, healthy diet

A healthy diet is an indispensable prerequisite for the use of aspecific micronutrient supply. Only with a balanced diet are the supplied micronutrients optimally absorbed by the gastrointestinal tract. Athletes do not automatically become Olympic champions through sports-scientific training, a balanced diet and the required targeted customized micronutrient supply. But it is also true that an optimal supply of micronutrients is proven to significantly reduce the high injury risk of competitive athletes (see pg. 100-102) and thus creates a training continuity that is urgently needed to achieve top performances.

Individual reactions are possible

Individual differences may occur in the athletes' reaction to a specific supply of a number of micronutrients such as, for instance, L-carnitine. We refer to *responders* and *non-responders*.

Basic supply only

Many previously offered commercial micronutrient products (various juice concentrates, powders, etc.) and recommended dosages are meant to serve as a basic supply but cannot meet the competitive athlete's individual requirements.

Product quality

Important information: Quality must be a consideration when choosing micronutrients. According to research at the Institute for Biochemistry at the German Sports Academy in Cologne, Germany, of 634 dietary supplements 94 (14.8%) tested positive for anabolic androgenic steroids (AAS).

Certified and tested quality

The customized micronutrient formulations shown here are based on the HCK® building block module product line. They are only available through pharmacies, AMSPORT and are subject to regular inspection via WADA anti-doping regulations and a few mono preparations.

8.4 Examples of micronutrient therapy for competitive athletes based on a balanced diet

SALUTO's database is the foundation for an optimal combination of customized micronutrients based on intracellular measurements of vitamins, minerals, and trace elements. Ascertaining the TSH-level (provides information about thyroid activity), measuring individual amino acids and the ferritin level are also essential for the preparation of the customized micronutrient formulation.

The combination of required micronutrients resulted primarily from the building block system as well as the AM-formula blend. Depending on blood test results, iron, magnesium or omega-3 fatty acids were given separately in individual cases.

About the micronutrients given to the competitive athletes

AM-formula blend (AMSPORT) is an enzymatic protein hydrolysate with short-chain peptides and L-amino acids of the highest purity and quality. Dosage recommendations were based on blood test results. Further details about the combination of individual amino acids can be found on page 99. We got exceptionally good blood test results in competitive athletes who took aspecific supply of this amino acid blend.

Optimal intake mode: 10 g before and 20 g diluted in a sports drink after each training session. Our regular nutrition analyses and blood tests of amino acids show that in spite of a balanced diet, professional team handball and soccer players have significant deficiencies which, among other things, have led to repeated problems in the tendon and ligament apparatus of these players. During intensive training and competition phases we recommend taking up to a maximum of 70 g over the course of the day. Avoid mixing with carbonated mineral water as this will considerably decrease the effectiveness.

The combination of customized micronutrient formulations for competitive athletes is based on cellular micronutrient analyses. A separate dose of iron was given in the form of *ferro sanol duodenal®*, as well as an additional dose of magnesium with magnerot classic® (orotate) 35 mg chewable tablets, if needed based on cellular blood tests.

In addition, in the evening athletes drank one half Kalinor effervescent tablet (from pharmacy) every day directly after training and competition phases and one half *Kalinor*® effervescent tablet in the evening, depending on blood test results.

High bioavailability

Balanced composition and bioavailability in the body are critical for the effectiveness of a micronutrient preparation. The body best absorbs micronutrients when they are embedded in plant cells like in fruits and vegetables. This is referred to as a *colloidal* state.

HCK® micronutrient granules are vitamins, minerals, trace elements, bioflavonoids and fiber that are embedded in a plant-based hydrocolloid (guarin, from guar). The resulting absorption-characteristics of the micronutrients are perfectly matched, as they would be in nature. The micronutrients embedded with the HCK®-method:

- guarantee optimal distribution pattern in the body,

- guarantee slow and gradual release from the gastrointestinal tract over a period of hours,

- prevent reciprocal interference between micronutrients,

- can be individually adapted to the micronutrient requirements of each athlete based on the intracellular micronutrient analysis, and

- reconciles vitamins, minerals, trace elements, bioflavonoids and fiber with each other.

Regular use of these customized micronutrient formulations can only work in conjunction with a balanced diet because an acidic metabolic status can significantly decrease the absorption of micronutrients (see pg. 219-227).

Measures of central tendency

Examined athletes (4,741 females and 4,409 males) consumed an average 3,195 ± 626 kcal. The results of the competitive athletes' nutrition analyses conformed up to 93% to the amounts recommended by the DGE for each respective athletic activity. The total energy supply was comprised of 57% carbohydrates, 26% fat, and 17% protein, which nearly meet recommendations. The average fluid supply was 4.5 ± 1.31 l. For most micronutrients the supply and routine serum blood tests were in a normal range, while cellular tests (in the erythrocytes) of micronutrients (Mg, Zn, Se, B_1, B_2, B_6, B_9) showed considerable deficiencies.

We will show what a customized micronutrient formulation for a particular athlete should look like based on the respective cellular blood test result, by means of individual examples from the entire spectrum of tested athletes.

Anthropometric data from 9,150 competitive athletes

	Age (years)	Height (cm)	Weight (kg)	BMI (kg/m²)
Total (N = 9,150)	26.3 ± 9.9	180 ± 4.5	71.45 ± 4.4	22.05
Female (N = 4,741)	24.3 ± 7.3	175 ± 4.3	68.1 ± 4.2	22.3
Male (N = 4,409)	28.2 ± 8.3	185 ± 4.8	74.8 ± 4.6	21.9

Distribution by sport

Soccer	Team hand-ball	Basket-ball	Tennis	Track & Field	Marathon	Triathlon	Other sports: race-runners, Martial arts (e.g. Judo), Cyclists, etc.
4,150	1,129	312	830	760	420	879	670

447 European junior national league players:
Germany/Netherlands/France/Spain
2,170 professional soccer players, 467 professional team handball players, 121 professional tennis players, etc.
89 Olympic champions/world champions/European champions (all sports)

Fig. 73

Micronutrient formulation for a 20-year old junior national team handball player leading up to a world championship victory 2008 in Egypt

Our lab physicians spoke of a latent thyroid hypofunction based on a borderline TSH-level of 4.2 µIU/ml (a TSH-level of > 2.8 can already result in increasing incidents of fatigue, night sweats and poor regeneration ability), which can lead to a considerable performance decrease in competitive athletes. (When ascertaining these levels a possible exertion-induced increase in thyroid hormone levels due to intensive training and playing on the previous day must be taken into consideration).

This player received 1.5 iodine tablets (Jodid 200) 10 minutes before breakfast. Regular follow-up thyroid hormone tests showed a definite return to normal levels (last TSH-level 1.9 µIU/ml). For this reason the micronutrient formulation based on the HCK® building block system does not contain iodine, because a separate supply in the morning before breakfast is more effective.

It has been our experience that the gastrointestinal system must get used to the micronutrient formulation dosages. Guar flour can initially cause some flatulence. The athlete therefore starts by taking only half the dose for one week, before taking the specified single dose of his personal formulation in the morning and at lunch with food.

On intensive training days the player also took up to 50 g of AMSPORT over the course of the day. 20 g directly after a training session to stabilize the various connective tissue structures (ligaments, tendons, various cartilage structures, etc.).

Table 11: Reference range of micronutrient concentrations with a customized micronutrient formulation

Customized micronutrient formulation for a 20-year old junior national team handball player (see criteria on pg. 171, fig. 72)			
Active ingredient per day	**Daily dose amount per 14 g**	**Active ingredient**	**Daily dose amount per 14 g**
Vitamins		**Trace elements**	
Vitamin A (retinol)	1 mg	Chromium	200 µg
Vitamin B$_1$ (thiamine)	30 mg	Manganese	10 mg
Vitamin B$_2$ (riboflavin)	30 mg	Molybdenum	100 µg
Vitamin B$_6$ (pyridoxine)	60 mg	Selenium	200 µg
Vit. B$_{12}$ (cyanocobalamine)	90 µg	Zinc	44 mg
Vitamin C (ascorbic acid)	1,500 mg	**Minerals**	
Vitamin D$_3$	15 µg	Calcium	200 mg
Natural Vitamin E	300 mg	Potassium	200 mg
From		Magnesium	200 mg
alpha tocopherol	254.7 mg	Silicium	20 mg
Gamma tocoperhol	40 mg	**Quasi vitamins**	
Natural carotinoids	8 mg	Choline	240 mg
From		Coenzyme Q$_{10}$	30 mg
alpha carotene	70 µg	Inositol	180 mg
Beta carotene	1.9 mg	L-carnitine	500 mg
Cryptoxanthine	15 µg	PABA	60 mg
Leutin	6.0 mg	**Plant extracts**	
Zeaxanthin	15.0 µg	Green tea extract	350.8 mg
Biotin (vitamin H)	100.0 µg	Citrus bioflavinoids	375.9 mg
Folic acid (vitamin B$_9$)	1.2 mg	Red wine extract	350.8 mg
Niacin (Vitamin B$_3$)	30 mg	**Fiber**	
Pantothenic acid	60 mg	Guar flour	3,585.7 mg
Daily intake mode: 3 scoops: 1.5 scoops morning and afternoon		HPM cellulose	139.6 mg
		Inulin	184.2 mg

Table 12: Amino acid concentration intake with daily dose of 50 g AMSPORT

Amino acid	Specifications for the intake of 50 g (AM-formula blend)
L-alanine	4.4
L-arginine	4.1
L-aspartic acid	3.0
L-glutamic acid	5.5
L-glycine	10.3
L-histidine	0.3
L-isoleucine	2.4
L-leucine	0.8
L-lysine	1.7
L-methionine	1.9
L-phenylalanine	1.1
L-proline	6.7
L-serin	1.6
L-threonine	0.9
L-tyrosine	0.2
L-valine	1.2

In the evening the player again took 5 x 35 mg *magnerot classic*® chewable tablets with food. Two hours before bedtime he took 2 x 500 mg tryptophan.

Micronutrient formulation dosages are checked 2-3 times each year and formulations are readjusted for the individual athlete.

Testimonial by the 20-year old junior world champion

"For the past year I have been injury-free for the first time in several years. Since SALUTO prepared the customized micronutrient formulation for me based on special intracellular blood tests and the regular intake of the AM-formula blend, my performance has increased significantly. I have been feeling much better since then. The optimal micronutrient supply proved to be a critical factor in the development of physical fitness (no training interruptions due to injury without external force) for many of my teammates and myself and resulted in our junior world championship-win in 2009."

Case study of the development of a top tennis talent from age 13 to age 17

- Amount of training: started with 14 hours of training at age 13 per week

- Current amount of training: 25-30 hours per week

- Initial situation: frequent infections, including Epstein-Barr virus (Pfeiffer glandular fever)

The tennis player came to us at age 13, after all other medical, clinical and advanced immunological tests did not produce any discernible information. During the previous weeks the very talented tennis player had barely been able to complete his training due to constant minor infections. He described:

- increased fatigue,

- certain amount of listlessness,

- some night sweats, and

- significantly longer regeneration period.

The results showed blatant deficiencies in the area of cellular micronutrient concentrations even though the athlete had already been taking specific micronutrients according to DGE guidelines. The nutrition analysis results were largely consistent with DGE specifications. Lowered ferritin levels of 32.1 ng/ml

Table 13

Micronutrient	Total active ingredient concentration	Morning	Afternoon	Evening
Magnerot Classic® (orotate) 1 tablet contains 35 mg magnesium	350 mg		5 x 35 mg	5 x 35 mg
Zinc histidine (gluconate)	45 mg	1 x 15 mg	1 x 15 mg	1 x 15 mg
Vitamin B complex, Taken in the course of the day	B-Vitamins (B_1 16,5 mg, B_2 19,5 mg, B_3 30 mg, B_6 21,5 mg, B_9 1.200 µg, B_{12} 90 µg)	2	3	
Vitamin C in depot form	2,000 mg	2 x 500 mg	2 x 500 mg	
Vitamin E Natural vitamin E	270 mg	1 x 270 mg		
Selenium (yeast bound)	150 µg	1 x 50 µg		2 x 50 µg
Omega-3 fatty acids (Ameu)	2.000	1 x 1,000 mg		1 x 1,000 mg
Iron *Ferrosanol duodenal®* 3 x a week, in the evening	100 g	1		
L-carnitine *L-carnipure*™	1,000 mg		1 x 500 mg	1 x 500 mg
Jodid 200 10 minutes before breakfast	200 µg	1,5		
Glutamine	3,000 mg			1 x
L-tryptophan	1,000 mg			2 x 500 mg

and borderline thyroid levels (basal TSH-level, T_3, T_4) also showed signs of a beginning hypofunction. Advanced immunological tests showed decreased phagocytic function ("eating ability of monocytes and granulocytes").

An all-day base-acid profile was done for three days each week (see pg. 226). Over the next four months the player received the following micronutrient formulation (see table). Since we did not yet use HCK® building block system supplements five years ago, this therapy was initially done with a variety of mono preparations primarily from commercial Taxofit products, at different times of the day. The major disadvantage of thatspecific customized micronutrient formulation was the great range of products the athlete had to take (in some instances up to 16 different tablets per day).

The competitive athlete also received 30 g of a high-quality amino acid blend as described on page 173, Table 9.

Due to the identified thyroid hypofunction the athlete was given 1.5 Jodid 200 tablets in the morning, 10 minutes before breakfast.

After four months, we performed another intracellular micronutrient blood test and also checked the immune system. The blood sample was taken after a three-day regeneration period.

Since the targeted use of the micronutrient supply the athlete did not have any infections and was able to complete the training program in optimal form. The significant decrease in phagocytic function of monocytes and granulocytes returned to normal. There verifiably was no evidence of any bacterial or viral infection at the time of either test.

Phagocytic activity at the beginning and after the four-month period:

• monocytes: (310-1,110) from 160.8 to 780.2

• granulocytes: (590-1,260) from 324.7 to 810.3

Since that time the development of the customized micronutrient formulation based on the building block system, a supply of 30 to 70 g of AM formula-blend, *L-thyroxine*[75]® due to an existing thyroid hypofunction, and regular use of iron (*ferro sanol duodenal*®) for curative purposes, have resulted in an optimal stability

Table 14

Customized micronutrient formulation for a 17-year old tennis player with a training volume of 28 hours a week (see criteria on pg. 171, fig. 72)			
Active ingredient per day	Daily dose amount per 16 g	Active ingredient	Daily dose amount per 16 g
Vitamins		**Trace elements**	
Vitamin A (retinol)	1 mg	Chromium	200 µg
Vitamin B$_1$ (thiamine)	40 mg	Manganese	10 mg
Vitamin B$_2$ (riboflavin)	40 mg	Molybdenum	100 µg
Vitamin B$_6$ (pyridoxine)	90 mg	Selenium	200 µg
Vit. B$_{12}$ (cyanocobalamine)	120 µg	Zinc	44 mg
Vitamin C (ascorbic acid)	2,500 g	**Minerals**	
Vitamin D$_3$	15 µg	Calcium	200 mg
Natural Vitamin E	300 mg	Potassium	400 mg
From		Magnesium	400 mg
alpha tocopherol	254.7 mg	Silicium	20 mg
Gamma tocoperhol	40 mg	**Quasi vitamins**	
Natural carotinoids	8 mg	Choline	240 mg
From		Coenzyme Q$_{10}$	30 mg
alpha carotene	70 µg	Inositol	180 mg
Beta carotene	1.9 mg	L-carnitine	1,000 mg
Cryptoxanthine	15 µg	PABA	60 mg
Leutin	6.0 mg	**Plant extracts**	
Zeaxanthin	15.0 µg	Green tea extract	350.8 mg
Biotin (vitamin H)	100.0 µg	Citrus bioflavinoids	375.9 mg
Folic acid (vitamin B$_9$)	1.2 mg	Red wine extract	350.8 mg
Niacin (vitamin B$_3$)	40 mg	**Fiber**	
Pantothenic acid	80 mg	Guar flour	3,585.7 mg
		HPM cellulose	139.6 mg
		Inulin	184.2 mg
Daily intake mode: 4 scoops: 2 scoops morning and afternoon		In addition to AMSPORT the amino acids	
		Glutamine	2,000 mg
		Arginine	2,000 mg

L-thyroxine 75® every morning before breakfastsince the athlete has a proven hypothyroid condition (hypofunction). *Ferro sanol duodenal®* 2-3 times per week in the evening with food, 5 x 35 mg additional supply of *magnerot classic®* chewable tablets two hours before bedtime; 2 x 500 mg tryptophan two hours before bedtime.

of the immune system in spite of a current training volume of up to 28 hours a week (at the tender age of 17). In addition, there were no more problems with the entire active and passive musculoskeletal apparatus (tendon, ligament apparatus).

Today the athlete receives customized micronutrient formulations based on the results of intracellular micronutrient tests, results from a nutrition analysis and an additional protocol sheet. The current formulation is as follows:

Table 15: Daily amino acid concentration supply ingested with a 50 g dose of AM-formula blend

Amino acid	Specifications for the intake of 50 g (AM-formula blend)
L-alanine	4.4
L-arginine	4.1
L-aspartic acid	3.0
L-glutamic acid	5.5
L-glycine	10.3
L-histidine	0.3
L-hydroxypoline	0.5
L-isoleucine	2.4
L-leucine	0.8
L-lysine	1.7
L-methionine	1.9
L-phenylalanine	1.1
L-proline	6.7
L-serin	1.6
L-threonine	0.9
L-tyrosine	0.2
L-valine	1.2

Case study of a top tennis player
(ranked among top-ten in the world)

The top tennis player described his last complete season as riddled with frequent infections, repeated minor injuries, especially to many connective tissue structures (ligaments, tendons, muscles), that prevented any kind of training continuity. In addition he felt physically and mentally exhausted. He trained for an average 30 hours a week. The results from the special blood test showed a latent thyroid hypofunction with an actual basal TSH-level of 3.4 µIU/ml.

The blood test was preceded by a two-day rest period, so that the effects of an intensive training session or competition on the thyroid hormones could be ruled out. In our experience, a TSH-level of 2.8 µIU/ml can lead to significant long-term adverse effects on physical and mental capacity. After an in-depth endocrinologic test the player received a separate iodine preparation (1.5 Jodid 200) in the morning, 10 minutes before breakfast. After as little as six weeks, the basal TSH-level returned to normal at 1.9 µIU/ml.

In addition his ferritin level of 35.6 mg/dl showed significant deficiencies for a competitive athlete (see pg. 134-136). The player received *ferro sanol duodenal®* for one month in the evening with food (less strain on the gastrointestinal system), and subsequently only twice a week. After only three months there was a distinct improvement of ferritin levels to 89.9 mg/dl.

The blatant deficiencies of micronutrients specifically amino acids to vitamins and trace element, were one of the primary causes for the many minor injuries to connective tissue structures. It was apparent that this athlete's micronutrient requirements increased considerably with an intensive training and competition workload, and that only a targeted micronutrient formulation can meet these requirements.

During the following season this top tennis player was able to fully meet his potential, establishing himself among the top-ten players in the world.

The player's customized micronutrient formulation was based on a special intracellular blood test, his nutritional results and the analysis of an attached log. This is what it looked like:

Table 16

Customized micronutrient formulation for a top tennis player with a training volume of 30 hours a week			
Active ingredient per day	**Daily dose amount per 16 g**	**Active ingredient**	**Daily dose amount per 16 g**
Vitamins		**Trace elements**	
Vitamin A (retinol)	1 mg	Chromium	200 µg
Vitamin B$_1$ (thiamine)	40 mg	Manganese	10 mg
Vitamin B$_2$ (riboflavin)	40 mg	Molybdenum	100 µg
Vitamin B$_6$ (pyridoxine)	90 mg	Selenium	200 µg
Vit. B$_{12}$ (cyanocobalamine)	400 µg	Zinc	44 mg
Vitamin C (ascorbic acid)	2,500 g	**Minerals**	
Vitamin D3	15 µg	Calcium	200 mg
Natural Vitamin E	300 mg	Potassium	400 mg
From		Magnesium	400 mg
alpha tocopherol	254.7 mg	Silicium	20 mg
Gamma tocoperhol	40 mg	**Quasi vitamins**	
Natural carotinoids	8 mg	Choline	240 mg
From		Coenzyme Q$_{10}$	60 mg
alpha carotene	70 µg	Inositol	180 mg
Beta carotene	1.9 mg	L-carnitine	1,000 mg
Cryptoxanthine	15 µg	PABA	60 mg
Leutin	6.0 mg	**Plant extracts**	
Zeaxanthin	15.0 µg	Green tea extract	350.8 mg
Biotin (vitamin H)	100.0 µg	Citrus bioflavinoids	375.9 mg
Folic acid (vitamin B$_9$)	1.2 mg	Red wine extract	350.8 mg
Niacin (vitamin B$_3$)	40 mg	**Fiber**	
Pantothenic acid	80 mg	Guar flour	3,585.7 mg
		HPM cellulose	139.6 mg
		Inulin	184.2 mg
Daily intake mode: 4 scoops: 2 scoops morning and afternoon		In addition to AMSPORT the amino acids	
		Glutamine	2,000 mg
		Arginine	3,000 mg

1.5 Jodid 200 tablets every morning before breakfast because the athlete has a proven hypothyroid condition (hypofunction). *Ferro sanol duodenal*® 2-3 times per week in the evening with food, an additional supply of 6 x 35 mg *magnerot classic*® chewable tablets two hours before bedtime. 1 x 500 mg tryptophan two hours before bedtime.

Table 17: The amino acid concentration taken daily for three months in a dose of 70 g AM-formula blend

Amino acid	Specifications for the intake of 70 g (AM-formula blend)
L-alanine	5.6
L-arginine	6.9
L-aspartic acid	4.0
L-glutamic acid	9.5
L-glycine	14.0
L-histidine	0.92
L-isoleucine	3.3
L-leucine	4.2
L-lysine	2.5
L-methionine	0.4
L-phenylalanine	1.4
L-proline	9.0
L-serin	1.2
L-threonine	1.3
L-tyrosine	0.70
L-valine	4.4

The development of the customized micronutrient formulation based on the HCK® building block system, a supply of 70 g AMSPORT, 1.5 Jodid due to an existing thyroid hypofunction, and a regular curative supply of iron (*ferro sanol duodenal®*), have since that time led to an optimal performance development in spite of a current training volume of up to 30 hours a week. There also were no more problems in the entire active and passive (tendon-ligament apparatus) musculoskeletal system. After three months we changed the composition of the customized micronutrient formulations in several areas.

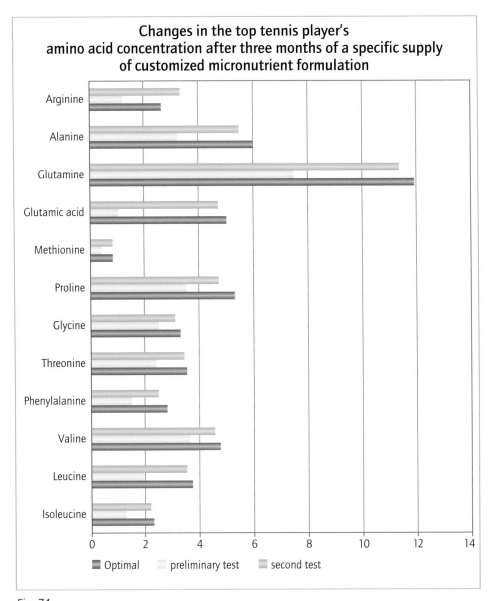

Fig. 74

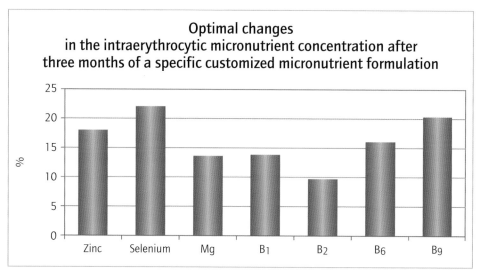

**Optimal changes
in the intraerythrocytic micronutrient concentration after
three months of a specific customized micronutrient formulation**

Fig. 75

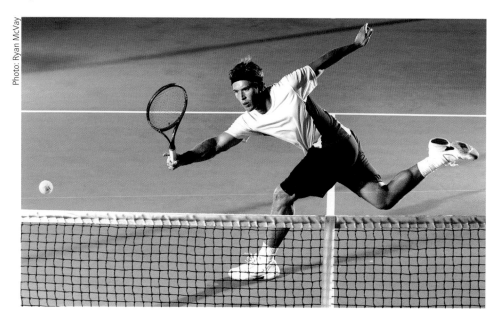

Photo: Ryan McVay

Case study of an Olympic champion and world champion in an endurance sport (5,000-10,000 m), training volume is 32 hours a week

The athlete exhibits a high susceptibility to infections during intensive training and competition phases.

193

This in particular interfered with his training continuity and thus the development of his optimal performance. The athlete described a certain amount of listlessness, insufficient regeneration after intensive training sessions, and many minor connective tissue injuries without external force (tendon-ligament apparatus, musculature).

All clinical/cardiological tests did not identify any further causes. A serologic test also (Western blot test) showed no abnormalities.

However, the results from the intracellular micronutrient analysis did show blatant deficiencies. An intracellular magnesium concentration of 36 mg/l Ery., a zinc concentration of 7, 7 mg/l Ery., a selenium concentration of 63 µg/l Ery., and marginal cellular B-vitamin concentrations are much too low for an endurance athlete to have a stable immune system. Chromium levels of 44 nmol/l signaled a very low full blood count. The results showed a slightly reduced specific cellular immunity. The blood test that was done after a three-day break from training showed no acute viral or bacterial infections at the time of the test and the blood count interpretation could thus proceed without restrictions.

Particularly obvious were the significant amino acid deficiencies (arginine, proline, methionine, and others) that are responsible for the stability and formation of the various connective tissue structures.

The results of the nutrition analysis showed a balanced diet in accordance with DGE (German Nutrition Society) guidelines.

We created the following micronutrient formulation (see table 18) with the aid of the intracellular micronutrient analysis, several additional blood parameters, the nutrition analysis evaluation and an additional protocol sheet. After a three-month regular supply this very successful athlete missed no more training sessions and was able to optimally develop his performance potential. Even the previously recurring minor injuries to the tendon-ligament apparatus and musculature were no longer detectable.

Important information: After three months, the formulation was changed in some areas due to a new intracellular micronutrient test.

Table 18

Customized micronutrient formulation for a former Olympic champion in an endurance sport with a training volume of 32 hours a week (see criteria on pg. 171, fig. 72)			
Active ingredient per day	Daily dose amount per 16 g	Active ingredient	Daily dose amount per 16 g
Vitamins		**Trace elements**	
Vitamin A (retinol)	1 mg	Chromium	200 µg
Vitamin B$_1$ (thiamine)	50 mg	Iodine	200 µg
Vitamin B$_2$ (riboflavin)	50 mg	Manganese	20 µg
Vitamin B$_6$ (pyridoxine)	100 mg	Molybdenum	200 µg
Vit. B$_{12}$ (cyanocobalamine)	200 µg	Selenium	200 µg
Vitamin C (ascorbic acid)	2,000 g	Zinc	44 mg
Vitamin D$_3$	15 µg	Copper	6 mg
Natural Vitamin E	300 mg	**Minerals**	
From		Calcium	200 mg
alpha tocopherol	254.7 mg	Potassium	400 mg
Gamma tocoperhol	40 mg	Magnesium	400 mg
Natural carotinoids	8 mg	Silicium	20 mg
From		**Quasi vitamins**	
alpha carotene	70 µg	Choline	400 mg
Beta carotene	1.9 mg	Coenzyme Q$_{10}$	90 mg
Cryptoxanthine	15 µg	Inositol	300 mg
Leutin	6.0 mg	L-carnitine	2,000 mg
Zeaxanthin	15.0 µg	PABA	100 mg
Biotin (vitamin H)	100.0 µg	**Plant extracts**	
Folic acid (vitamin B$_9$)	1.2 mg	Green tea extract	350.8 mg
Niacin (vitamin B$_3$)	50 mg	Citrus bioflavinoids	375.9 mg
Pantothenic acid	100 mg	Red wine extract	350.8 mg
		Fiber	
		Guar flour	3,585.7 mg
		HPM cellulose	139.6 mg
		Inulin	184.2 mg
Daily intake mode: specified number of scoops: Taken in the morning and afternoon		In addition to AMSPORT the amino acids	
		Glutamine	3,000 mg
		Arginine	2,000 mg

* An additional supply of 8 x 35 mg *magnerot classic*® chewable tablet with dinner. 3 x 1,000 mg omega-3 fatty acids; 2 x 500 mg tryptophan two hours before bedtime.

Table 19: The amino acid concentration that was given daily for three months with the supply of 70 g AM-formula blend.

Amino acid	Specifications for the intake of 70 g (AM-formula blend)
L-alanine	5.6
L-arginine	6.9
L-aspartic acid	4.0
L-glutamic acid	9.5
L-glycine	14.0
L-histidine	0.92
L-isoleucine	3.3
L-leucine	4.2
L-lysine	2.5
L-methionine	0.4
L-phenylalanine	1.4
L-proline	9.0
L-serin	1.2
L-threonine	1.3
L-tyrosine	0.70
L-valine	4.4

Case study of a 23-year old top professional soccer player

The top pro-soccer player described frequent minor injuries during the previous season, particularly to many connective tissue structures (ligaments, tendons, musculature) resulting in a lack of training continuity. He also felt physically and mentally exhausted. His average training volume was 20 hours a week. The special blood test results showed a latent thyroid hypofunction with current basal TSH-level of 3.8 µIU/ml. The blood test was preceded by a two-day rest period, so

Table 20

Customized micronutrient formulation for a top soccer player with a training volume of 20 hours a week (see criteria on pg. 171, fig. 72)			
Active ingredient per day	**Daily dose amount per 16 g**	**Active ingredient**	**Daily dose amount per 16 g**
Vitamins		**Trace elements**	
Vitamin A (retinol)	1 mg	Chromium	150 µg
Vitamin B$_1$ (thiamine)	30 mg	Manganese	15 mg
Vitamin B$_2$ (riboflavin)	30 mg	Molybdenum	150 µg
Vitamin B$_6$ (pyridoxine)	60 mg	Selenium	150 µg
Vit. B$_{12}$ (cyanocobalamine)	90 µg	Zinc	36 mg
Vitamin C (ascorbic acid)	1,500 g	**Minerals**	
Vitamin D$_3$	15 µg	Calcium	200 mg
Natural Vitamin E	300 mg	Potassium	400 mg
From		Magnesium	400 mg
alpha tocopherol	254.7 mg	Silicium	20 mg
Gamma tocoperhol	40 mg	**Quasi vitamins**	
Natural carotinoids	8 mg	Choline	240 mg
From		Coenzyme Q$_{10}$	60 mg
alpha carotene	70 µg	Inositol	180 mg
Beta carotene	1.9 mg	L-carnitine	1,000 mg
Cryptoxanthine	15 µg	PABA	60 mg
Leutin	6.0 mg	**Plant extracts**	
Zeaxanthin	15.0 µg	Green tea extract	350.8 mg
Biotin (vitamin H)	100.0 µg	Citrus bioflavinoids	375.9 mg
Folic acid (vitamin B$_9$)	1.2 mg	Red wine extract	350.8 mg
Niacin (vitamin B$_3$)	30 mg	**Fiber**	
Pantothenic acid	60 mg	Guar flour	3,585.7 mg
		HPM cellulose	139.6 mg
		Inulin	184.2 mg
Daily intake mode: 1.7 scoops: morning and afternoon		In addition to the AM-formula blend the amino acid	
		Arginine	3,000 mg

1.5 Jodid 200 tablets every morning before breakfast because the athlete has a proven hypothyroid condition (hypofunction). *Ferro sanol duodenal®* 2-3 times per week in the evening with food, an additional supply of 6 x 35 mg *magnerot classic®* chewable tablets two hours before bedtime.

Table 21: The amino acid concentration that was given daily with the supply of 50 g AM-formula blend.

Amino acid	Specifications for the intake of 50 g (AM-formula blend)
L-alanine	4.4
L-arginine	4.1
L-aspartic acid	3.0
L-glutamic acid	5.5
L-glycine	10.3
L-histidine	0.3
L-hyroxypoline	0.5
L-isoleucine	2.4
L-leucine	0.8
L-lysine	1.7
L-methionine	1.9
L-phenylalanine	1.1
L-proline	6.7
L-serin	1.6
L-threonine	0.9
L-tyrosine	0.2
L-valine	1.2

* 1 x 500 mg tryptophan two hours before bedtime.

that any impact on thyroid hormones from an intensive training session or competition could be ruled out. In our experience a TSH-level of 2.8 µIU/ml can have a significant long-term adverse effect on physical and mental capacity. After an in-depth endocrinological test the payer received a separate iodine preparation (1.5 Jodid 200) in the morning 10 minutes before breakfast. After only six weeks the basal TSH-level returned to normal at 2.0 µIU/ml.

In addition his ferritin level of 40.6 mg/dl showed considerable deficiencies for an endurance athlete (see pg. 134-136). The player received *ferro sanol duodenal*® (less strain on the gastrointestinal system) in the evening with dinner for one month, and after that only twice a week. There was a definite improvement in his ferritin level to 80.9 mg/dl after only three months.

The blatant deficiencies in the area of micronutrients from amino acids all the way to vitamins and trace elements are one of the primary causes of the many minor connective tissue injuries. It became apparent once again through this athlete, that intensive training and competition workloads clearly increase micronutrient requirements and that only a specific micronutrient formulation can meet these requirements.

During the following season this top soccer player was able to meet his full performance potential and over the following two years showed no signs of injuries without external force.

The player's customized micronutrient formulation was based on a special intracellular blood test, his nutritional results and the analysis of an attached log (see table 20 and 21).

Case study of a performance-oriented endurance athlete, training volume 8-12 hours

The endurance athlete described frequent minor injuries during recent years, particularly to various connective tissue structures (ligaments, tendons, musculature) resulting in a lack of training continuity.

The athlete shows obvious signs of increased fatigue and poor regeneration ability. The results from the nutrition analysis show a balanced diet in accordance with German Nutrition Society guidelines. The average training volume was 8-12 hours per week. The results from the special blood test showed a basal TSH-level of 1.9 µIU/ml. In our experience a basal TSH-level of > 2.8 µIU/ml can lead to significant long-term adverse effects on physical and mental capacity. This could be ruled out with this athlete.

In addition his ferritin level of 41.6 mg/dl showed considerable deficiencies for an endurance athlete (see pg. 134-136). The player received *ferro sanol duodenal*®

Table 22

Customized micronutrient formulation for anendurance athlete with a training volume of 8-12 hours a week (see criteria on pg. 171, fig. 72)			
Active ingredient per day	**Daily dose amount per 16 g**	**Active ingredient**	**Daily dose amount per 16 g**
Vitamins		**Trace elements**	
Vitamin A (retinol)	1 mg	Chromium	100 µg
Vitamin B$_1$ (thiamine)	20 mg	Manganese	10 mg
Vitamin B$_2$ (riboflavin)	20 mg	Molybdenum	100 µg
Vitamin B$_6$ (pyridoxine)	40 mg	Selenium	100 µg
Vit. B$_{12}$ (cyanocobalamine)	60 µg	Zinc	36 mg
Vitamin C (ascorbic acid)	1,000 g	**Minerals**	
Vitamin D$_3$	15 µg	Calcium	200 mg
Natural Vitamin E	300 mg	Potassium	200 mg
From		Magnesium	300 mg
alpha tocopherol	254.7 mg	Silicium	20 mg
Gamma tocoperhol	40 mg	**Quasi vitamins**	
Natural carotinoids	8 mg	Choline	160 mg
From		Coenzyme Q$_{10}$	30 mg
alpha carotene	70 µg	Inositol	120 mg
Beta carotene	1.9 mg	L-carnitine	250 mg
Cryptoxanthine	15 µg	PABA	40 mg
Leutin	6.0 mg	**Plant extracts**	
Zeaxanthin	15.0 µg	Green tea extract	350.8 mg
Biotin (vitamin H)	100.0 µg	Citrus bioflavinoids	375.9 mg
Folic acid (vitamin B$_9$)	800 µg	Red wine extract	350.8 mg
Niacin (vitamin B$_3$)	20 mg	**Fiber**	
Pantothenic acid	40 mg	Guar flour	3,585.7 mg
Daily intake mode: split specified number of scoops: morning and afternoon		HPM cellulose	139.6 mg
		Inulin	184.2 mg
		Arginine	2,000 mg

* *Ferro sanol duodenal*® 2-3 times per week in the evening with food, an additional supply of 5 x 35 mg *magnerot classic*® chewable tablets two hours before bedtime.

Table 23: The amino acid concentration that was given daily for three months with a supply of 30 g AM-formula blend

Amino acid	Specifications for the intake of 50 g (AM-formula blend)
L-alanine	2.4
L-arginine	2.8
L-aspartic acid	1.7
L-glutamic acid	4.1
L-glycine	6.0
L-histidine	0.4
L-isoleucine	1.40
L-leucine	1.8
L-lysine	1.1
L-methionine	0.2
L-phenylalanine	0.6
L-proline	3.84
L-serin	0.5
L-threonine	0.5
L-tyrosine	0.3
L-valine	1.9

* 500 mg tryptophan in the evening two hours before bedtime.

(less strain on the gastrointestinal system) in the evening with dinner for one month, and after that only three times a week. There was a definite improvement in his ferritin level to 80.9 mg/dl after only three months.

The blatant deficiencies in the area of micronutrients from amino acids all the way to vitamins and trace elements are one of the primary causes of the many minor connective tissue injuries. It became apparent once again through this athlete, that intensive training and competition workloads clearly increase micronutrient

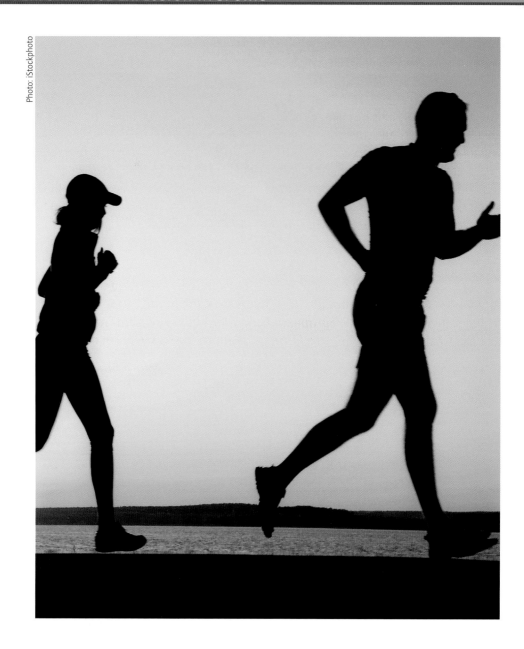

Photo: iStockphoto

requirements and that only a specific micronutrient formulation can meet these requirements.

In subsequent years the endurance athlete was able to meet his whole performance potential and showed no signs of connective tissue injuries.

Development of a micronutrient concentration for youth national league players leading up to the European championship win in 2008

The following two illustrations (Fig. 77, 78) show the efficient development of a cellular micronutrient concentrationwith individual doses of HCK® micronutrient formulations prepared according to the individual player's requirements based on blood tests, nutrition analyses and an additional protocol sheet (see pg. 171, Fig. 72). Dosages correspond to the formulations described on pages 181-200. Additional doses of iron in cases of low ferritin levels, omega-3 fatty acids and separate doses of magnesium were given.

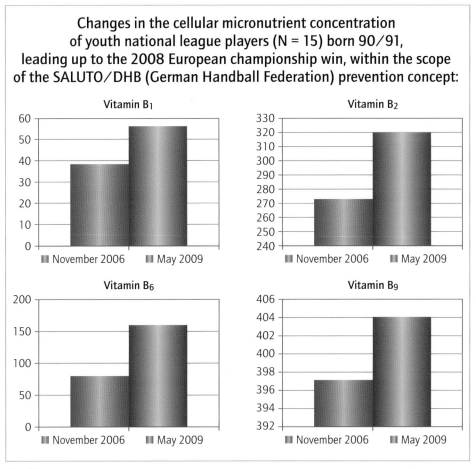

Changes in the cellular micronutrient concentration of youth national league players (N = 15) born 90/91, leading up to the 2008 European championship win, within the scope of the SALUTO/DHB (German Handball Federation) prevention concept:

Fig. 76

In addition to the HCK® micronutrient formulations players received doses of 30 to 70 g of the AM-formula blend over the course of the day. Dosages of high-quality amino acids are based on blood test results and the player's diet.

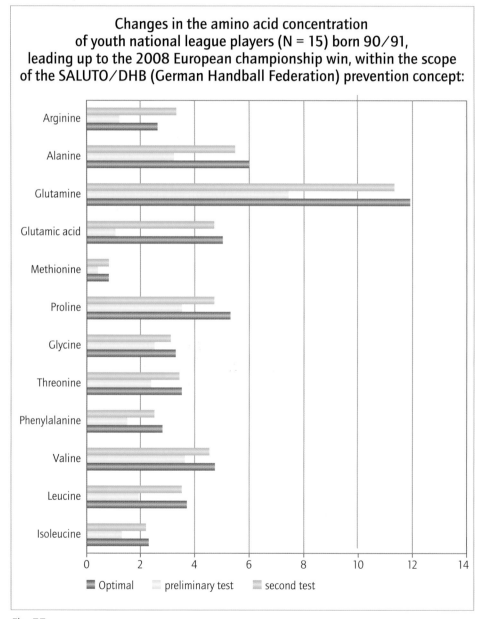

Fig. 77

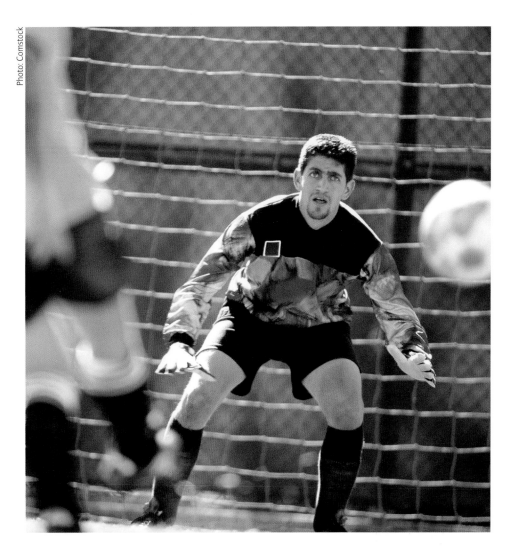

Photo: Comstock

Development of a micronutrient concentration for junior national league players leading up to the world championship win in 2009

The following two illustrations (Fig. 79 and 80) show the efficient development of a cellular micronutrient concentration with individual doses of HCK® micronutrient formulations prepared according to the individual player's requirements based on blood tests, nutrition analyses and an additional protocol sheet. Dosages correspond to the formulations described on pages 181-200. Additional doses of iron in cases of low ferritin levels, omega-3 fatty acids and separate doses of magnesium were given.

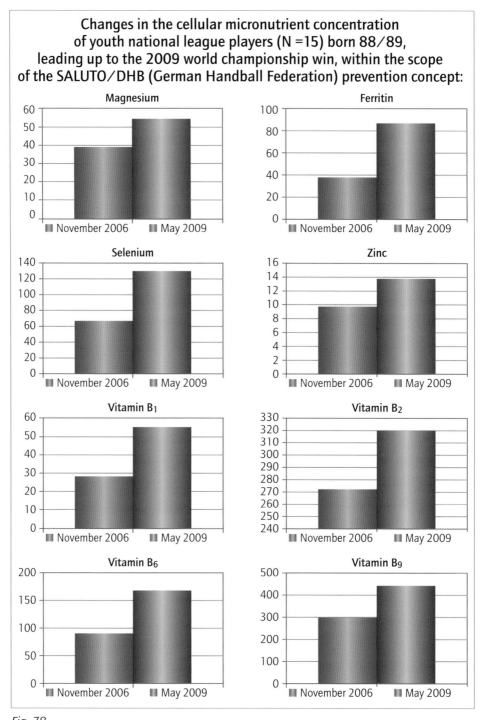

Changes in the cellular micronutrient concentration
of youth national league players (N =15) born 88/89,
leading up to the 2009 world championship win, within the scope
of the SALUTO/DHB (German Handball Federation) prevention concept:

Fig. 78

In addition to the HCK® micronutrient formulations players received doses of 30 to 70 g of the AM-formula blend over the course of the day. Dosages of high-quality amino acids are based on blood test results and the player's diet.

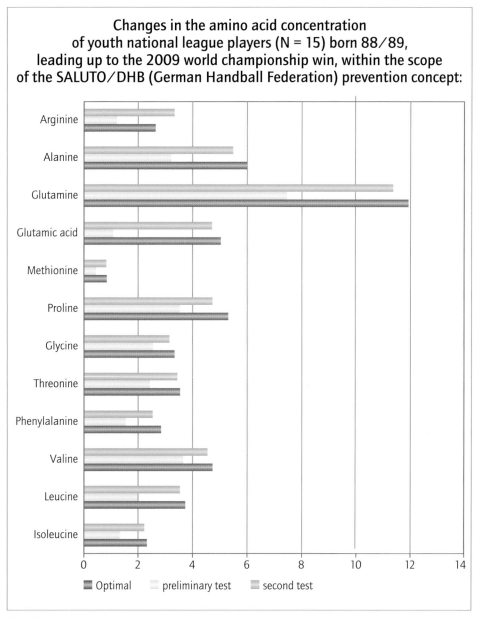

Fig. 79

Development of a micronutrient concentration for 1,150 athletes over a four-month period

(comparison with customized micronutrient formulation and DGE dosage recommendations along the lines of German Society for Sports Medicine/Prevention)

The anthropometric data and results from nutrition analyses of both groups are listed on pages 100-102. These differ only slightly in the two groups and are in line with DGE guidelines. Optimal effects of the cellular micronutrient concentrations are evident in the competitive athletes (N = 559) (see table 24) who took specific customized micronutrient formulations (dosage recommendations as described on pages 181-200). This is also reflected in a very low infection rate in the immunological tests.

After four months of intensive training and competition phases, the other group of athletes (N = 591) who regularly took micronutrients based on previous DGE dosages showed a noticeably increasing deficiency (see table 25).

Tab. 24: Development of intraerythrocytic micronutrient concentration zinc, magnesium, selenium, B-vitamins (B_1, B_2, B_6, B_9) in competitive athletes (N = 559) taking customized doses of micronutrient formulations according to specifications from intracellular blood tests over a period of time (comparison between start of preparatory phase and after four months).

	Unit	Prelim. test	Exit test	Δ%
Zn (**)	mg/l Ery.	9.0 ± 1.1	12.4 ± 1.4	+ 27.4
Se (**)	µg/l Ery.	80.3 ± 12.1	103.5 ± 12.9	+ 12.4
Mg (**)	mg/l Ery.	41.2 ± 4.2	46.1 ± 5.0	+ 6.8
B_1 (**)	µg/l Ery.	39.8 ± 11.8	62.9 ± 12.5	+ 36.7
B_2 (**)	µg/l Ery.	312.2 ± 39.2	399.7 ± 34.1	+ 21.9
B_6 (**)	µg/l Ery.	40.1 ± 13.8	69.9 ± 13.0	+ 42.6
B_9 (**)	µg/l Ery.	189.2 ± 63.2	273.8 ± 78.9	+ 31.9

Tab. 25: Development of intraerythrocytic micronutrient concentration zinc, magnesium, selenium, B-vitamins (B₁, B₂, B₆, B₉) in competitive athletes (N = 591) according to previous dosage recommendation guidelines by the German Society for Sports Medicine and Prevention over a period of time (comparison between start of preparatory phase and after four months).

	Unit	Prelim. test	Exit test	Δ%
Zn (**)	mg/l Ery.	9.8 ± 1.3	8.0 ± 1.6	− 18.4
Se (**)	µg/l Ery.	88.3 ± 10.1	68.5 ± 9.9	− 22.4
Mg (**)	mg/l Ery.	44.2 ± 5.2	38.1 ± 3.9	− 13.8
B₁ (**)	µg/l Ery.	41.8 ± 13.8	35.9 ± 8.5	− 14.1
B₂ (**)	µg/l Ery.	332.2 ± 30.2	299.7 ± 30.1	− 9.8
B₆ (**)	µg/l Ery.	44.1 ± 10.8	36.9 ± 10.0	− 16.3
B₉ (**)	µg/l Ery.	193.2 ± 60.2	153.8 ± 58.9	− 20.4

In addition the N = 559 competitive athletes received a supply of the AM-formula blend (30 to 70 g per day) depending on blood test guidelines, nutrition analysis and protocol sheetresults.

The other group of competitive athletes (N = 591) did not receive a separate supply of amino acids in accordance with previous DGE and German Society for Sports Medicine and Prevention guidelines. The following illustration also shows that the intensive training and competition phase lead to a significant drop in this group's amino acid concentration (see pg. 211, Fig. 81).

The rate of injuries without external force in this group is, as described on page 101, considerably higher. Connective structures in particular require a specific supply of these micronutrients to stabilize ligaments, tendons and musculature. This produces new findings for the future that also require more long-term scientific testing with appropriate MRT imaging. The relationship between a sufficient micronutrient supply and susceptibility to infection and injury can be proven. However, previous results also show that dosage recommendations by the DGE and the DGSP (German Society for Sports Medicine and Prevention) must be critically examined.

Changes in intraerythrocytic micronutrient concentrations

▌▌ Supply of **personalized doses of micronutrient formulations** in accordance with intracellular blood testspecifications, results from the nutrition analysis, the protocol sheet, and the criteria listed on pg. 171, fig. 72 for N = 559 competitive athletes.

▌▌ Dosage recommendations based on previous guidelines of the DGE and the **German Society for Sports Medicine and Prevention** for N = 591 endurance athletes.

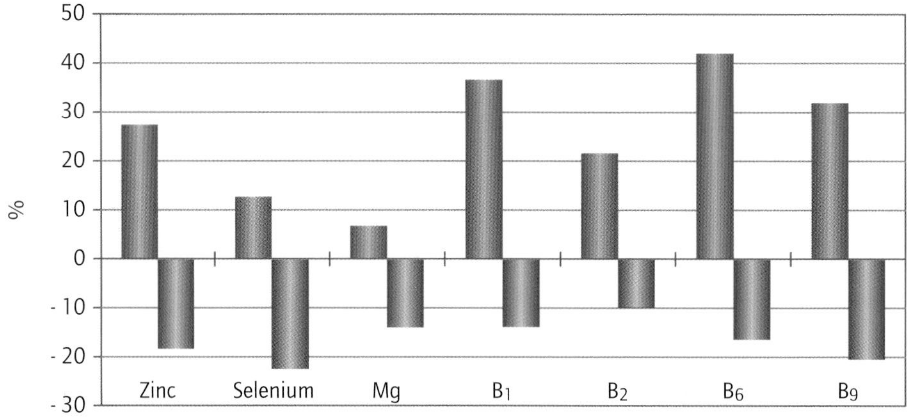

Time of first measurement: Start of the preparation phase
Time of second measurement: after four months

Fig. 80

To date sports medicine lacks exercise physiology data for the practical examination of the clinical relevance of previous dosage recommendations. The previously recommended supply is based purely on basic considerations regarding the relationship between energy use and increased nutrient requirements. This clearly requires some catching up over the next few years.

The increased high-quality amino acid requirements in the competitive athletes who did not take a supply of amino acids during intensive training and competition phases (over a period of four months) are shown in the Fig. 81. A specific supply of 30 to 70 g of an amino acid blend resulted in a verifiable improvement of the amino acid concentration and in conjunction with the customized micronutrient formulation, verifiably reduced the risk of injury without external force.

Changes in some amino acid concentrations

■ With a supply of AM-formula blend (30 to 70 g as required) depending on blood test specifications, results from the nutrition analysis, the protocol sheet, and the criteria listed on pg. 171, fig. 72 for N = 559 endurance athletes.

■ No separate supply of amino acids based on the **previous guidelines of the DGE and the German Society for Sports Medicine and Prevention** for N = 591 endurance athletes.

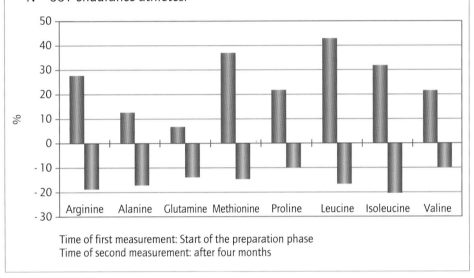

Time of first measurement: Start of the preparation phase
Time of second measurement: after four months

Fig. 81

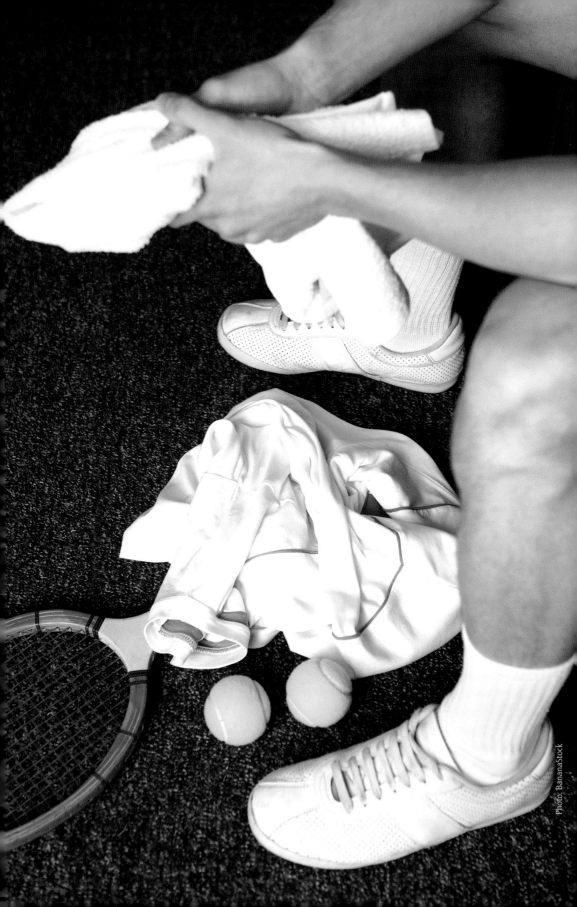

9 Optimal nutrition and performance enhancing wellness – references and tips

9.1 Fluid balance in athletes – optimal, intelligent and effective

Sweat loss is often underestimated in sports. Timely hydration is critical to athletic performance because even a fluid loss in sweat (dehydration) of only 2% of body weight can severely decrease performance. The perspiration rate depends on body weight, and the intensity and volume of athletic exertion. The higher the body weight and the higher the intensity and outside temperature, the higher the sweat loss.

The onset of dehydration (fluid deficit) impairs temperature regulation and diminishes the athlete's performance. When adequately hydrated body temperature as well as heart rate are considerably lower during exertion.

Table 26: Sweat loss in runners (ml per hour)

Degree of exertion%	Weight (kg)	10° C (ml)	15° C (ml)	20° C (ml)	25° C (ml)	30° C (ml)
70	60	770	770	930	1,095	1,260
70	70	945	945	1,120	1,295	1,470
85	60	1,020	1,020	1,195	1,370	1,545
85	70	1,250	1,250	1,440	1,525	1,815

Compiled from Friedrich, Optimale Sporternährung

Consequences of dehydration

The negative impact of insufficient hydration becomes already apparent at the first signs of thirst, with a slowly rising heart rate due to the blood's increasing viscosity (equals 1% loss of starting weight). A water deficit already causes a slight decrease in athletic performance. There are some simple behavioral rules to help the athlete maintain performance stability.

Sweating during physical activity protects from life-threatening overheating *(hyperthermia)*. But no loss of nutrients causes a drop in performance as quickly as water loss (dehydration) because our cells are no longer receiving sufficient amounts of oxygen and nutrients. The results are dizziness, muscle cramps and circulatory problems. For this reason the athlete must learn to drink enough before, during and after exercise.

Caution: Fluid intake should be increased gradually so gastrointestinal receptors can get used to increased amounts of fluid; otherwise the athlete will quickly feel unwell (feeling bloated).

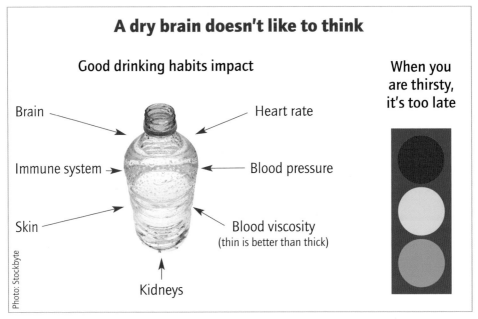

Fig. 82

Fluid intake during moderate endurance workloads

The maximal fluid intake per hour is limited by the speed of gastric emptying. Maximal fluid passage from the stomach for beverages is between 1,000 and 1,200 ml per hour, whereby these numbers decrease considerably at an intensity of more than 70% of maximal performance. For a moderate endurance workload it is recommended to drink 250 ml of fluid every 15 minutes.

Fluid intake during intensive endurance workloads

During intensive endurance workloads the speed of gastric emptying is considerably slower. This means less fluid is transported to the intestine and the blood. Liquid intake during intensive endurance workloads should be only 4 x 150-200 ml per hour. During multiple hour endurance workloads fluid intake should therefore begin after only 30 minutes of exertion. The table clearly shows that we lose more sweat than we can absorb in fluids, making dehydration inevitable.

Important information

Research shows that during intensive exertion endurance athletes often drink less than half of the recommended amount of 600-800 ml per hour. Consequently dehydration in athletes causes a much quicker drop in performance.

Quick fluid passage from the stomach through effective drinking

The following factors facilitate quick fluid passage from the gastrointestinal tract:

- 6-8% percent carbohydrates in beverages (equals 60-80 g carbohydrates per liter).

- Avoiding apple or orange juice in competitive sports during intensive exertion; this inhibiting effect on gastric empting also occurs when mixing apple juice with equal amounts of mineral water.

- Timely hydration is important because gastric emptying slows down considerably toward the end of the exertion period due to already existing dehydration.

- Avoiding liquid portions of more than 500-600 ml; optimal fluid intake is 250 ml every 15 minutes after initial 30 minutes.

- Drinking hypotonic (highly concentrated) beverages.

Isotonic and hypotonic beverages ensure effective drinking

Beverages with a high percentage of carbohydrates (dextrose, fructose) have many individual particles. These beverages have a higher number of particles than blood and are therefore hypertonic. When Colas or fruit beverages are consumed the mucous membranes in the gastrointestinal tract must first release water to dilute these beverages. This is particularly undesirable during exertion because it causes fluid loss in the intestinal mucous membranes. The number of individual particles is much smaller when using maltodextrin. It makes the beverage isotonic (same number of particles as blood) or hypotonic (lower particle concentration than blood). Isotonic or hypotonic beverages are better suited for quick fluid replacement in sports because mucous membranes in the gastrointestinal tract do not have to release additional water for dilution.

Optimal choice – mineral water with a high percentage of hydrogen carbonate

The effects of a sufficient bicarbonate concentration (hydrogen carbonate) on performance during intensive and highly intensive exertion have been scientifically proven for a long time. A sufficient supply of bicarbonate in particular reduces the drop of lactic acid, decreases subjective fatigue during identical workload intensity, and increases performance during highly intensive workloads, lasting until exhaustion.

Athletes with highly intensive workloads should choose beverages high in bicarbonate (mineral water containing minimum 50mg/l, optimal > 1,500 mg/l bicarbonate, if possible before, but also during athletic exertion to increase the blood's acid-buffering capacity. By increasing the bicarbonate reserve in the blood (HCO_3-reserves) the muscle is able to deliver the accrued acid (H+) to the blood. The muscle is able to neutralize more quickly and thus becomes efficient again. The bicarbonate (HCO_3) can then absorb the muscle's acid, thereby creating carbonic acid (H_2CO_3). Carbonic acid breaks down into carbon dioxide (CO_2) and water (H_2O) and is exhaled through the lungs. Next to a high percentage of hydrogen carbonate, sodium content of > 350 mg/l is also critical.

A good sodium balance is absolutely necessary during multiple hour exertion

The most important mineral on a quantity basis that is lost when sweating, is sodium. 1l of sweat contains an average 1 g of sodium.

Athletes acclimatized to heat lose less sodium in sweat (0.5 g per 1l sweat). An unfit runner who is not acclimatized to heat loses considerably more sodium 1.8 g per 1l sweat). A slight sodium deficiency due to sweat loss can easily develop during longer, multiple hour exertion, particularly during warmer temperatures. The effects of sodium deficiency (hyponatremia) are initially muscle cramps and muscle stiffness.

Important information

People who experience a constant urge to urinate during multiple hour endurance workouts should add more sodium (2 g salt per beverage) to a beverage before and during exertion because sodium binds more strongly with water in the body. This can slow down elimination via the kidneys. It is important to remember that an increased urge to urinate with higher consumption of tea or drinking water during multiple hour exertion is caused by the low sodium content.

Sodium supply during extended athletic endurance workloads

- Cramping during athletic exertion can only be alleviated with sodium.

- Taking magnesium during athletic exertion is counterproductive because magnesium can cause stomach cramps and even diarrhea.

- During multiple hour endurance workouts sodium content in mineral water should be at least 450 mg sodium per liter up to 1,000 mg sodium per liter.

- The amount of sodium ingested with solid food after athletic exertion is not sufficient because it comes too late.

Summarizing charts on this topic (see appendix) can be downloaded as a PDF-file from the publisher's website with the user name "explosion" and the following code number: xutRZ4qt

Keeping a drinking log is helpful

No other loss of nutrients decreases performance as quickly as a water deficiency (dehydration) because our muscle cells are no longer getting a sufficient supply of oxygen and nutrients. It therefore makes sense to keep a daily drinking log. A master copy of the drinking log (see appendix pg. 278) can also be downloaded as a PDF-filefrom the publisher's website with the user name "explosion" and the following code number: xutRZ4qt

The following example shows how expedient such a log can be:

M. Mustermann drinking log

Date	Time	Quantity	Beverage	Location
03.12.07	7 am	0.3 l	fruit tee	hotel
	9 am	0.5 l	water/juice	hotel
	noon-3 pm	0.7 l	juice & water mix	home
	5 pm-7 pm	0.5 l	mineral water	car
	8 pm	0.3l	beer	home

Important:
Weight **before** training (without clothing)
Weight **after** training (without clothing)

Add an **additional 0.5 l** drink requirement to the weight difference.

Example:
89 kg before training, 87 kg after training =
2 kg difference = 2 l + 0.5 l = 2.5 l
Drink requirement in addition to basic requirement is 2 l.

Fig. 83

9.2 Optimal base-acid ration ensures good micronutrient absorption

The anti-doping concept with customized micronutrient therapy for competitive athletes only makes sense in conjunction with a balanced diet. If the athlete thinks he can compensate for his "poor" eating habits with the customized micronutrient formulations shown here, he will fail. Optimal absorption of the required micronutrients can only take place in a good base-acid environment.

Prosperity creates acidity

Today most people, but especially competitive athletes from industrialized nations have a diet that is too "sour". Base foods are on the menu too seldom or in small amounts. People in postindustrial nations live better than ever, at least with regard to nutrition and way of life. Many of our health problems today are associated with the prosperity factor *hyperacidity*, which is linked to an endless number of illnesses including muscle aches, joint rheumatism, chronic fatigue, an overall weakened immune system, etc.. Even teeth are affected because the acidic saliva attacks the enamel and no longer supplies enough micronutrients to repair the damage. Hyperacidity can generally be considered a creeping widespread disease. It usually remains undetected for many years, unlike the suddenly occurring life-threatening hyperacidity of a diabetes patient, called *acidosis*. The human organism has the ability to balance the impact of organic acids for a long time before it sounds the alarm through illness.

But we have good news: You can continue to eat whatever you like without restriction. But you should make sure that the proportions are correct. The formula is simple: Eat four times as many base foods as acidic ones.

What causes hyperacidity?

Foods and stimulants produce acid in the body. The metabolism for instance, generates carbonic acid in all of the body's cells. The breaking down of animal proteins, but also plant proteins, generates phosphoric and sulfuric acid in the metabolism. This effect is intensified by stress, lack of exercise or, in competitive athletes, intensive training sessions.

Acids and bases

Acid sensitivity varies greatly in humans. The so-called ph-level with a scale of 5.2 to 7.4 was introduced to visually measure this subjective sensitivity, whereby ph-levels of 5.2 to 6.5 are considered acidic and ph-levels of 6.8 to 7.5 are primarily base.

Slag accumulates

Acids are necessary for the body's energy production. But an excess of acids causes the metabolic processes to "foam over". Preferable is the balance between the two opposites, the acid-base balance. As long as the body does not generate or intake sufficient amounts of base bicarbonate, only a portion of these undesirable substances is transformed into an excretable substance. The remainder of the dissolved slag is in a way just rearranged. Removed from one place it is redeposited in another.

Competitive athletes are often diagnosed with hyperacidity

We have already illustrated basic links between cellular micronutrient deficiencies and degenerative changes in many connective tissue structures (tendon, ligament apparatus, cartilage structures) (see page 105-109). In addition to the listed micronutrient deficiencies that share in the responsibility for increasing hyperacidity in competitive athletes, this hyperacidity in the form of "acidic nutrition" also accelerates degenerative changes of the cartilage matrix. The thickened synovial fluid mixed with salt crystals forms a gelatinous matter that wears away cartilage matrix with each movement. Softer and more pliable bones from many years of demineralization facilitate this process.

A balanced diet based on DGE (German Nutrition Society) criteria is the most important foundation for an optimal base-acid ratio.

Balancing hyperacidity naturally

Normally the human organism balances the formation of the previously mentioned acids without any problems. The body has various protective mechanisms and buffer systems to withstand damaging hyperacidity as long as possible. In doing so ituses minerals obtained from plant-based foods. But if the diet contains too few of these base substances the acids that form are temporarily stored primarily in connective tissue, but later also in muscles and joints. While connective tissue can tolerate relatively large amounts of the mentioned acids, blood is particularly acid-sensitive. Higher acid content makes the transport of vital oxygen from the lungs to the cells more difficult. The body tries to manage this by extracting calcium from the bones to neutralize the acid that is forming.

Beneficial counterforce – base nutrition

The human body generates acid, and does so in excessive amounts, if it has an imprudent diet. It receives base substances exclusively from the outside, mostly from plant-based foods. Someone who eats plenty of potatoes, root, bulb, herbaceous and leaf vegetables, or various types of fruits has a base diet. There is a very simple rule of thumb for maintaining an acid-base balance: eat four times as many base foods as acidic foods. That means less meat, fish, eggs, dairy products, but lots of vegetables of any kind, fruit, potatoes, whole grain pasta and rice. Fats are acid neutral but make you gain weight, which is why they should be approached with caution.

How do I recognize acidosis (hyperacidity)?

Later on we will provide a detailed demonstration of how do perform a three-day acid-base profile test. The following complaints are associated with hyperacidity:

- weakened immune system, constant colds or lingering infections,

- digestive problems with constipation or chronic irritable bowel syndrome with bloating,

- acid regurgitation or gastritis,

- constant cold feet or hands,

- hard or tense muscles, particularly in the neck, shoulder and back,

- highly stressed nervous system, irritability and fatigue,

- pain of the skin or the entire body, chronic pain that goes undiagnosed even after intensive diagnostic evaluations.

Water – a barrier against hyperacidity

Drinking sufficient amounts of the right fluids is very important to your health: next to plant-based foods water or mineral water are the best suppliers of base minerals; carbonic acid is harmless and is quickly exhaled through the lungs.

Mineral water should be very high in hydrogen carbonate (HCO_3). Any water containing more than minimum 500mg/l, optimal 1500 mg/l (HCO_3) is recommended for competitive athletes. Calcium content should be higher than 150 mg/l, magnesium more than 50 mg/l.

In addition:

- Alcohol should only be consumed in small amounts.

- Coffee consumption should be moderate as it promotes calcium excretion.

- Beverages containing sugar should be crossed off the grocery list. Instead purchase unsweetened fruit juices, herbal teas and vegetable juices.

Acids and bases in our food

The body's natural acid-base ratio is approximately 1:4. To achieve this ratio we really only need to know what produces acids and bases. This becomes obvious after only a short period of time. Many acid producers can be replaced by healthier foods. For example, substitute polished rice with much tastier unpeeled rice.

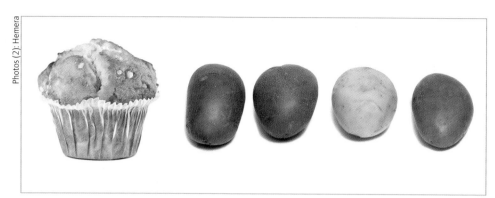

Fig. 84: Optimal base-acid ratio

Important information

For competitive athletes: White pasta and white rice are favorites. Try to eat mostly whole grain pasta and/or wild rice on training days because they do not produce excessive amounts of acid. But do not eat whole grain pasta (rice) on competition days because they stay in the gastrointestinal tract too long.

We differentiate between four basic food groupswith respect to their impact on the body's acid-base balance:

Base-producing foods

These include primarily:

- potatoes,
- vegetables,
- herbs, such as parsley, chives, marjoram, thyme, paprika, dill, oregano,
- fruit
- raw milk and
- uncarbonated mineral water.

Neutral foods

These maintain acid-base equilibrium. They include:

- butter,

- walnuts,

- natural plant oils and

- tap water.

Acid producers

These are foods that do not contain acids themselves, but generate them during metabolic breakdown:

- sugar,

- sweets containing sugar (marzipan, chocolate, cake, ice cream),

- all peeled or polished grains and their products, also rye bread,

- soft drinks containing sugar, white flour products (rolls, white bread, pasta, dumplings, polished rice),

- coffee and

- alcoholic beverages.

Acid suppliers

These are protein-containing foods that supply large amounts of acidic minerals (sulfur, phosphorus, iodine, chlorine, etc.) Their consumption can produce additional acid during metabolism. Excessive meat consumption thereby doubles the base loss.

These include:

- meat and organ meats (liver, heart, kidneys, brains),

- poultry (chicken, duck, goose, turkey),

- game (rabbit, venison, wild boar),

- eggs (only the yolk is base),

- cheese, curds and

- meat broth.

Healthy acid-base balance

An optimal acid-base balance ensures absorption of customized micronutrient formulations. The acid-base balance can be measured with a simple three-day profile. You can measure your own profile with the aid of ph-test strips. These test strips along with the respective color chart can be found in any pharmacy.

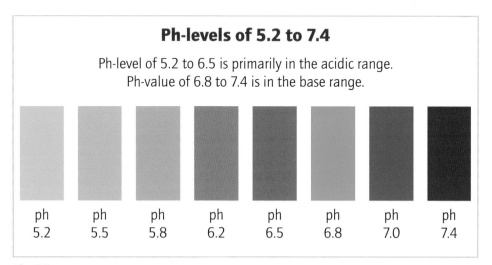

Ph-levels of 5.2 to 7.4

Ph-level of 5.2 to 6.5 is primarily in the acidic range.
Ph-value of 6.8 to 7.4 is in the base range.

| ph 5.2 | ph 5.5 | ph 5.8 | ph 6.2 | ph 6.5 | ph 6.8 | ph 7.0 | ph 7.4 |

Fig. 85

For this analysis the athlete receives a three-day protocol sheet. The ph should be measured in the morning on an empty stomach, in the afternoon and the evening before eating. It would be best if the athlete could collect a urine sample in a small container, dip the test strip in the urine for one second and then record the results based on the color chart. If the urine cannot be collected in a container the test strip can be briefly held in the urine stream and the results then recorded with the aid of the color chart. In addition, keep a record of the way you feel analogous to the protocol sheet.

You can download these protocol sheets from the publisher's website as a PDF-file using the user name "explosion" and the code number xutRZ4qt and enter your respective values. We recommend doing the protocol only on weekdays since diets tend to be slightly different on weekends.

Tab. 27: ACID-BASE PROFILE ph-test

First name/Last name: _____

	Day 1	Day 2	Day 3
In the morning before breakfast			
Physical condition			
Mental state			
Before lunch			
Physical condition			
Mental state			
In the evening before dinner			
Physical condition			
Mental state			

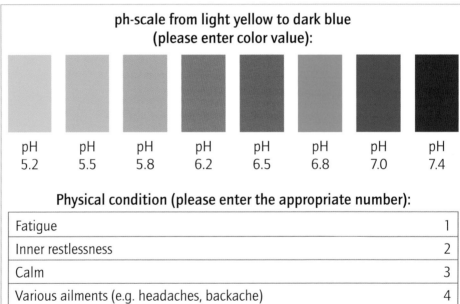

ph-scale from light yellow to dark blue (please enter color value):

| pH 5.2 | pH 5.5 | pH 5.8 | pH 6.2 | pH 6.5 | pH 6.8 | pH 7.0 | pH 7.4 |

Physical condition (please enter the appropriate number):

Fatigue	1
Inner restlessness	2
Calm	3
Various ailments (e.g. headaches, backache)	4
Muscle tightness	5
Active in sports	6

Mental state (Please enter a definition):

e.g. well, slept badly, even-tempered, stressed, etc.

Fig. 86: protocol sheet

Optimal balance of the base-acid ratio

Due to intensive physical exertion, the metabolism of competitive athletes is often in an acidic statein spite of a balanced diet.

If the results from the ph-test indicate an acid state of the metabolism we recommend a regular supply with a high-quality base powder. Depending on tolerability of the gastrointestinal tract, the athletes take a powder blend in the evening for a therapeutic effect. During intensive training phases it may be expedient to take it twice. It contains a synergetic blend of minerals and trace elements, as well as enzymes. It also improves the effectiveness of enzymes in the body (digestion and metabolism).

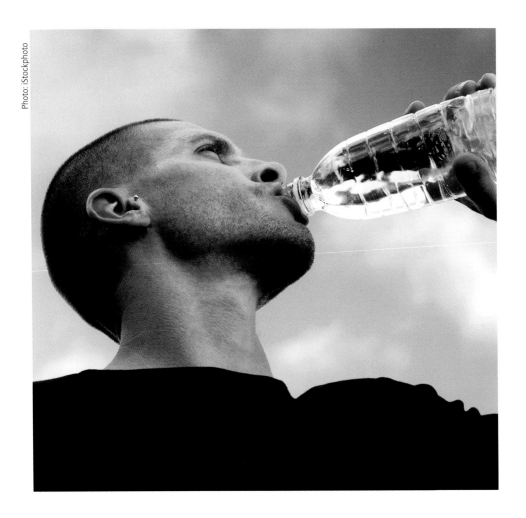

Photo: iStockphoto

Criteria for a health-conscious diet

- Choose foods (see pg. 219-227) that ensure an optimal base-acid ratio.

- Sufficient amounts of fluid ensure long-term performance. Choose mineral water low in carbonic acid and high in hydrogen carbonate > 1,500 mg (additional information on pg. 213-218).

- Learn to let your gastrointestinal receptors get used to the increased amount of fluids or you will frequently feel unwell.

- Keep a daily drinking log (see pg. 278).

- Eat lots of fresh fruits and vegetables during the day. Freshly pressed fruit and vegetable juice also count as fresh food portions.

- Reduce so-called *hidden fats from* sausage, cheese, sweets, desserts etc., and pre-made food products.

- Use plant-based oils high in unsaturated fats (e.g. rapeseed oil, cold-pressed olive oil).

- Increase your intake of ocean fish high in omega-3 fatty acids (halibut, salmon) to 2-3 times a week. If you really don't care for this, a minimum of 500 mg omega-3 fatty acids in the form of salmon oil capsules from a pharmacy would be sensible.

- Eat high-quality, lean, free-range meats (venison, poultry)

- Eat whole grain products high in fiber and minerals instead of micronutrient-poor white flour products.

- Handle foods with care to prevent further loss of micronutrients (example: steam vegetables briefly, otherwise too many vital nutrients are lost).

- Reduce alcohol consumption to a minimum (alcohol after intensive training significantly lengthens regeneration).

- Reduce cooking salt consumption to 5-6 g per day. Use iodized salt.

9.3 Optimal carbohydrate strategy – super-carbo-loading

Carbohydrate storage in the body

Carbohydrates are stored in the muscles and liver in the form of glycogen. Sufficiently full carbohydrate stores (glycogen stores) equal greater athletic capacity (see pg. 79-88, Energy Supply). If glycogen stores are not at optimal capacity from nutrition, structural proteinsbecome the primary source for energy production, and thus are no longer sufficiently available to stabilize the many connective structures, thereby verifiably significantly increasing risk of injuries without external force.

The glycogen repositories in the muscles are important for muscular work while the carbohydrates that are stored in the liver are needed to maintain a constant blood sugar level. All organs receive their energy supply via the blood sugar level. Stored carbohydrates must first be transformed into glucose (dextrose) before the muscles and the other organs can use them. Since the brain depends on a constant supply of dextrose from the blood, a severe drop in the blood sugar level can cause a lack of mental efficiency. In extreme cases athletes may experience a loss of balance and sudden dizziness.

An unfit person can store approximately 400 g of carbohydrates in the form of glycogen. Approximately 100g of these are in the liver and approximately 300 g are stored in the muscles.

Greater energy storage through a specific diet high in carbohydrates

Carbohydrates should make up the bulk of daily food intake. The carbohydrate portion of the total energy consumption should be approximately 60%. Our experiences in recent years show that the carbohydrate portion of the overall energy consumption of competitive athletes in particular is frequently only 45%. Preferred carbohydrates should be complex, long-chain and high-quality carbohydrates (pasta, bread, potatoes, rice, cereal).

Most important are complex carbohydrates (whole-grain products) instead of too much white pasta or rice, which will cause hyperacidity (see pg. 219-227).

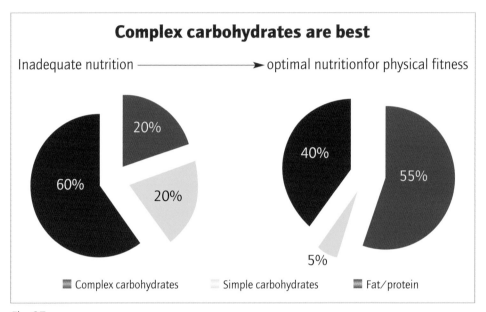

Fig. 87

The Fig 88 shows that competitive athletes often eat too many simple, empty carbohydrates that make up approximately 20% of the total diet. For long-term replenishment of glycogen stores in the liver and muscles, they should be at approximately 55%.

The goal: Multiple complex carbohydrates in the form of whole-grain products

Many competitive athletes prefer primarily white pasta, white rice and such. Although the carbohydrate content of refined carbohydrates is not lower they do, as previously mentioned, lead to a metabolism-related hyperacidity.

Natural carbohydrates have a much higher vitamin, mineral and trace element content than refined carbohydrates and contain considerably more fiber for healthy action of the bowels and healthy intestinal flora. Natural carbohydrates are also filling and are therefore not consumed in excessive amounts. The following information should be taken into consideration when consuming complex carbohydrates:

Tips for more carbohydrates

- Increase side dishes (whole grain products: pasta, rice, potatoes, bread).
- Reduce meat and fatty sauces.
- Cut bread slices thicker and reduce topping.
- Limit consumption of soft drinks.
- Fewer sweets.
- Desserts in the form of fresh fruit.

Fig. 88

The following illustration shows a list of foods containing complex carbohydrates that should be consumed more frequently:

Particularly whole-grain pasta, whole-grain rice, whole-grain bread, and potatoes are the types of carbohydrates that should make up the bulk of a meal.

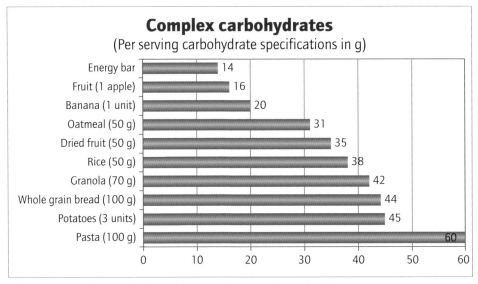

Fig. 89: compiled from DGE nutrition panel, 43rd edition, 2005

A breakfast high in carbohydrates

Mix a cereal from:

- 5 Tbsp Quaker oats (rolled Oats, whole-grain cereal)
- 3 Tbsp wheat germ
- 1 banana, sliced
- yoghurt (also vanilla yoghurt)

Serve with a glass of fresh-squeezed orange juice.

Optimal energy storage
through training and a specific carbohydrate supply

Athletic training initially depletes glycogen stores. Subsequent food intake that is high in carbohydrates replenishes glycogen stores beyond the original level. Competitive athletes who eat a diet high in carbohydrates therefore have greater energy reserves than people who do not exercise or eat fewer carbohydrates.

Carbohydrate stores and amount of energy as related todiet in competitive athletes compared to unfit individuals		
	Without training with a normal mixed diet	Through training with a diet high in carbohydrates
Blood sugar	5 g (20 kcal)	5 g (20 kcal)
Liver glycogen	75 g (300 kcal)	120 g (480 kcal)
Muscle glycogen	300 g (1,200 kcal)	500 g (2,000 kcal)
Total	380 g (1,520 kcal)	625 g (2,500 kcal)

Fig. 90: compiled from DGE nutrition panel, 43rd edition, 2005

Amount of carbohydrates needed for endurance training

This should be (according to Maughan et al, 2004) for:

- less than 10 hours, 5-7 g per kg of body weight/per day,
- more than 10 hours, 8-10 g per kg of body weight/per day.

An insufficient supply of carbohydrates increases the metabolization of important amino acids (arginine, methionine, proline, and others). For this reason a supply of high-quality carbohydrates is fundamental to the function of the energy metabolism and injury prevention.

An optimal micronutrient supply ensures good carbohydrate storage

Next to a supply of complex carbohydrates, a sufficient potassium and chromium supply is critical to good glycogen storage (carbohydrate storage) in muscles and liver. Additional information can be found in the chapter "Tasks and functions of individual micronutrients" (see pg. 131-164). Fruits and vegetables are especially high in potassium and should be eaten throughout the day. A sufficient chromium supply is important for the maintenance and replenishment of carbohydrate stores. A lack of chromium can severely inhibit replenishment of glycogen reserves.

Also important: Ingesting sufficient amounts of sodium through fluids in sports facilitate:

*   rapid carbohydrate absorption,

*   rapid water absorption, and

*   low urinary excretion.

Improved regeneration through a combination of carbohydrates and protein

Combining carbohydrates and protein results in quicker carbohydrate storage, within just a few hours, than carbohydrates alone. For this reason the first meal, or rather first beverage of a regeneration phase should contain not only carbohydrates, but also proteins.

A brief summary of the most important practical nutrition tips can be found in the appendix. These can be downloaded from the publisher's website as a PDF-file using the user name "explosion" and the following code number: xutRZ4qt

Optimal carbohydrate strategy – super-carbo-loading

Effective, modern carbo-loading includes food combinations that are high in carbohydrates, potassium and chromium while also supplying protein. These food combinations are particularly advisable on the last few days before a competition and immediately after training and competing.

The bulk of the energy contained in super-carbo-loading menus should always come from carbohydrates. The carbohydrate component should always be dominant in the make-up of these menus. In addition complex carbohydrates should largely be of the whole-grain variety. White pasta, white rice, etc., should only be eaten on competition days since whole-grain products to linger in the body due to their fiber content.

Nothing works without carbohydrates!

Food combinations that contain carbohydrates, potassium, and chromium while also supplying protein

Super-carboloading

Carbohydrate-rich foods	Potassium-rich foods	Chromium-rich foods	Protein-rich foods
Pasta	tomato soup	mushrooms	cheese, low fat
Rice	vegetables	mushroom gravy	peas, turkey
Bread	tomatoes, peppers	Edam cheese	cheese, low fat
Potatoes	curd cheese	Edam cheese	curd cheese, low fat, egg
Granola	fruit	whole grain cereal, Nuts	milk, yoghurt, low fat

Fig. 91: from Feil / Wessinghage "Ernährung und Training" (Nutrition and Training)

> **Note:**
> Use the accompanying diagram to create a personal food combination
>
> **Super-carboloading:**
> - It is important that carbohydrates dominate
> - Carbohydrates should come from whole grains: whole grain pasta, whole grain rice, whole grain bread
> - Please do not consume whole grain pasta/rice etc. on competition days (white pasta, etc. is easier digestible by the gastrointestinal system)
> - Organic produce: using potato peel – optimal for connective tissue formation

Fig. 92

9.4 Beneficial food combinations containing proteins

Next to a specific supply of customized amino acid dosages that are necessary for the stability and function of many connective tissue structures (ligaments, tendons, cartilage) (see pg. 85-97) a balanced, high-quality diet is a basic prerequisite for the health of competitive athletes.

A protein's biological valence stems from an amino acid pattern and specifies how much autologous protein can be formed from 100 g of nutritional protein.

The higher the essential (vital) amino acid content of a protein the more of it can be converted to autologous protein. Reference value here is a whole egg, which covers the daily requirements of an adult with 0.5 g per kg of body weight. Its biological valence is 100 (see Fig. 94).

In principal animal protein is of higher quality than plant protein, with the exception of amaranth (grain of the Inca), which has a higher biological protein valence than cheese and milk. Amaranth (available in health food stores) in particular, can be sprinkled on cereal in the form of popped amaranth seeds, and next to high-quality amino acids it also contains high-quality carbohydrates.

The single source protein with the highest biological valence of 104 is whey protein. A combination of plant and animal proteins can combine the nutritional proteins in their protein pattern intoa high-quality protein. A mix of whole egg and potatoes has the highest biological valence of 136.

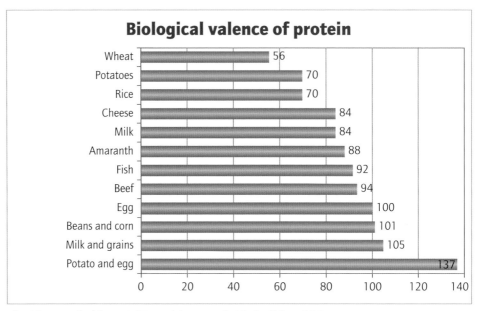

Fig. 93: compiled from DGE nutrition panel, 43rd edition, 2005

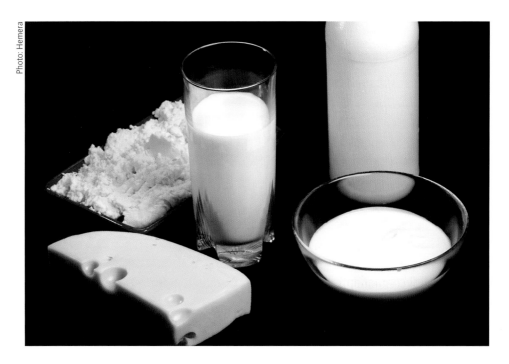

Beneficial combinations of foods containing proteins are recommended during the regeneration phase (see the following Fig. 94).

Other beneficial food combinations from the protein group

Grains with milk products
- Granola with milk or yoghurt
- Whole grain bread with cheese
- Pasta with cheese

Grains with legumes
- Beans with pasta, rice or potatoes
- Peas with pasta, rice or potatoes

Grains with eggs
- Pancakes, waffles

Potatoes with egg or milk products
- Unpeeled boiled potatoes with curd cheese
- Unpeeled boiled potatoes with fried egg
- Potatoes with cheese

Fig. 94

9.5 Foods containing silica are optimal nutrients for connective tissue structures

Amino acids and foods that contain silica (e.g. whole-grain products, horsetail extract, etc.) are the most important nutrients for strong connective tissue, and thus strong tendons and ligaments.

Silica's central componentis *silicon*. Silicon promotes the body's own production of collagen fibers and the matrix. Silicon also facilitates better cross linkage. Silica preparations are not recommended because absorption in the intestine is less than 1%, while nearly 100% of a watery horsetail extract is used.

Connective tissue stability reduces injury susceptibility

Impact of a diet that is high in silica:
- Resilience of tendons, ligaments and cartilage
  - Good wound and bone healing ability
    - Strong bone structure
  - Strengthens immune system

Foods that are high in silica:
- Common horsetail extract
  - Whole grain rice
    - Oatmeal
      - Millet
      - Barley
    - Potato peel

Fig. 95

9.6 A sound sleep ensures performance

Sufficient amounts of sleep ensure optimal recuperation after intensive training sessions or competitions especially for competitive athletes. Next to quality of sleep the regeneration of the intervertebral discs, among others, is crucial for competitive athletes. High-quality sleep reduces the release of stress hormones (cortisol) in competitive athletes.

Human growth hormone – the most important hormone at night

During the night our body switches to a different work mode whose objectives are rest and recuperation rather than performance. During the night an entire orchestra of hormones is busy getting us fit for the next day: The human *growth hormone* (HGH) is the most important hormone of the night. It promotes the production of new cells we need every day, provides energy-supplying substances such as fatty acids from fatty tissue, and breaks down the body's waste or slags.

This hormone in particular is very important to an athlete's ability to recuperate. At the onset of sleep the pituitary gland begins to produce the growth hormone. This production only ceases in the second half of the night during which we no longer have an actual deep sleep phase. The anabolic counteraction (rebuilding of structural proteins) after intensive training or competition is particularly important to long-term optimal performance development. Next to an optimal micronutrient supply, quality of sleep is the deciding factor in regeneration.

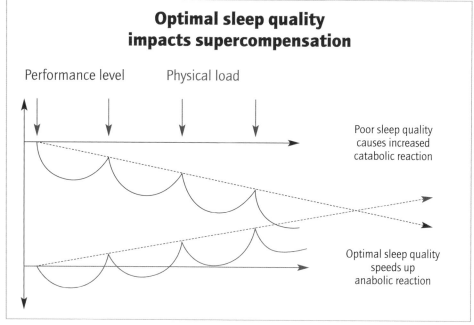

Fig. 96

The importance of cortisol as a regulating stress hormone

Cortisol is barely detectable during the first half of the night. From approximately 3:00 AM until morning, the cortisol level rises significantly, regardless of whether we are asleep or not. This hormone is directly controlled by the internal clock. Even if you don't go to sleep until 2:00 AM, the body begins to produce cortisol around 3:00 AM. With the onset of increased cortisol production the release of human growth hormone from the first half of the night is suspended, the blood sugar level rises, protein turnover and thus the metabolism are activated. In addition the

239

immune system, which was previously able to do its nightly work at top capacity without disruption, is suppressed. An excessive release of cortisol causes the opposite of restful sleep.

Someone who sleeps too little during the second half of the night, voluntarily or involuntarily, significantly increases his cortisol level, until it is so high that the athlete feels distressed. On the other hand, a high level causes us to sleep poorly and continue to wake up. Poor sleep quality during the first half of the night allows the cortisol level to rise considerably, eliminating any chance of restful sleep. This is fundamentally important for regeneration or rather the development of physical performance, particularly in competitive athletes.

Important information

A high-quality mattress or sleep surface verifiably reduces cortisol release. Based on our experiences and measurements of stress hormones in saliva, competitive athletes who slept on viscoelastic material experienced clearly better sleep quality. Competitive athletes take the opportunity to bring one of these flexible mattress pads in a bag to out-of-town training or competitions.

Create a relaxing sleeping environment

The illustration shows that competitive athletes who slept on the high-tech innovation pressure-relieving mattress pads developed by *Tempur®* for NASA's space program, exhibited a much lower cortisol release the following morning than the competitive athletes who had slept on a standard spring mattress.

The media maintains that turning over frequently during the night is an optimal way to regenerate the intervertebral discs. A collaborative study between competitive athletes and a sleep clinic show that, on the contrary, regeneration of the intervertebral discs (disci intervertebrales) does not depend on the frequency of turning over during the night but rather just the horizontal position.

Conclusion: Improved sleep quality (characterized by reduced cortisol release) leads to more rapid replenishment of depleted glycogen stores in the liver and

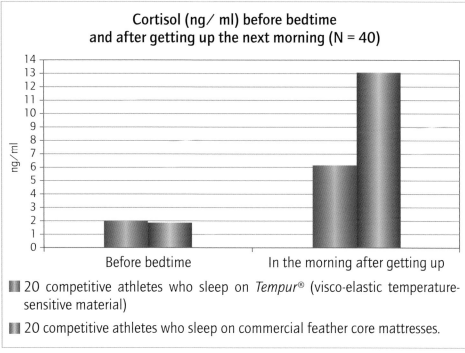

Fig. 97

muscles, and thus improved conditions for physical performance during the next training session or competition.

9.7 Achieve top-performance with proper BISA vibration training (biomechanical activation of the metabolism)

In recent years, vibration training has acquired cultural character. A lot of scientific research verifies the effectiveness of vibration training in elite sports, in the area of prevention and rehabilitation for improved quality of life.

The physiological mechanisms of optimal regeneration ability, strength development and muscular capacity through biomechanical stimulation (BMS) described by Nazarov, are present:

- in the optimization of inter and intramuscular coordination of muscle activity (stimulaton of mechanoreceptors of working muscles); nearly no involvement of passive musculature. In its reaction the organism therefore focuses all possible reserves on the muscles that are stimulated the most (dominance principle).

- in increased blood circulation, also resulting in more rapid removal of metabolites and faster supply of nutrients and oxygen to the muscle. This doubtlessly affects the effectiveness of training.

- in possible changes to muscle biochemistry that require further research.

The quality of the vibration technique is very important. Long-term use, especially in elite sports, but also in rehabilitation, can verifiably result in degenerative changes to many connective tissue structures (ligaments, tendons, cartilage).

Multidimensional vibration pattern – three-dimensional training

This is where most vibration technology manufacturers differ. In recent years we, of SALUTO, have had exceptionally positive experiences with the Innoplate vibration generator from SALUSSTAR® with vertical as well as diagonal vibrations, which offers a broad selection of training and therapy options. Particularly the unique vertical, diagonal and multidimensional waves with integrated oval. The diagonal mode corresponds to the natural motion patterns (walking, running).

Vibration via up-and-down movement, such as the vertical mode, does not have a tilt effect on the pelvis and thus no appreciable impact on the muscles of the back and pelvic floor. The maximum frequency at which the muscle is still able to react to every impulse is approximately 28 Hertz (vibrations per second).

Most scientific studies were conducted with frequencies of up to 30 Hertz. We have definite health-related concerns with frequencies higher than 35 Hertz. Preliminary tests show that exceeding these frequencies can accelerate long-term risk of degenerative changes of many connective tissue structures.

Improved regeneration ability in competitive athletes through specific BISA vibration training in addition to an optimal micronutrient supply

Rapid regeneration ability of the vegetative nervous system is crucial to the performance of athletes. The faster glycogen stores are replenished the more quickly the body regenerates and the sooner the body is ready for the next exertion. Tests performed by SALUTO show the impact of sports-related physical stress on the hormonal system. Multiple stresses (mental and physical) cause the stress hormone level to rise. One study with top athletes and 30 competitive athletes showed an increase in cortisol levels of up to 1,380% after intensive athletic exertion. A high cortisol level is proven to, among other things, severely inhibit replenishment of glycogen stores in liver and muscles after athletic exertion.

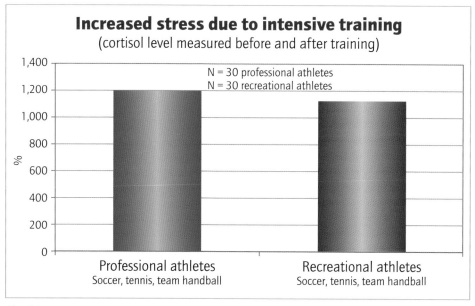

Increased stress due to intensive training
(cortisol level measured before and after training)

N = 30 professional athletes
N = 30 recreational athletes

Professional athletes
Soccer, tennis, team handball

Recreational athletes
Soccer, tennis, team handball

Fig. 98

Biomechanical stimulation with the aid of BISA vibration training by SALUSSTAR® Innoplate facilitates an increase in blood circulation, rapid removal of metabolites, accelerated supply of nutrients as well as improved supply of oxygen to the muscles. Vibration training has proven to accelerate cortisol breakdown and thus recuperation after intensive exertion. However, an insufficient supply of micronutrients inhibits the efficiency of BISA training.

Background knowledge

Cortisol is one of the body's most important hormones. It is produced in the adrenal cortex under influence of the brain (hypothalamus) and the pituitary gland (hypophysis). Unlike adrenaline, the body builds up a supply of cortisol, mainly (as previously described on pg. 240) during the second half of the night. Between 7:00 AM and 8:00 AM it is at maximum readiness for the day's activities. Cortisol levels drop sharply throughout the day, especially during the late morning. Only 10% of the morning's levels remain in the evening. The normal cortisol concentration in saliva is subject to dynamic fluctuations. Normal cortisol levels are between 5-15 ng/ml in the morning, while the levels drop to 0.3-3 ng/ml in the late afternoon and evening. Cortisol is not subject to relevant age-specific changes. Intensive physical and mental exertion can cause cortisol levels to rise significantly.

Case study – 26-year old competitive athlete, BMI (body mass index) 23.7

This competitive athlete has an optimal basic supply of micronutrients and an unremarkable basal TSH-level (also see pg. 146-150). A performance test helped us determine the individual aerobic-anaerobic threshold of 4.1 m/s and the fixed threshold (4 mmol/l) of 4.38 m/s. Cortisol release is measured with two tests within a three-day period. The athlete runs for 45 minutes at a predetermined

Tab. 28: Cortisol trend in a 26-year old competitive athlete with and without regenerative BISA training

	Running speed	Lactate after exertion mmol/l	Cortisol ng/ml before running	Cortisol ng/ml directly after exertion	Cortisol ng/ml after 15 minutes	Cortisol ng/ml after 45 minutes
With BISA Training	4.1 m/s	4.8	2.5	6.6	4.9	2.2
Without BISA Training	4.1 m/s	4.5	2.3	6.4	7.9	7.9

speed within the individual threshold area. Cortisol levels are measured before, immediately after running, after 15 minutes and after 45 minutes. After the first test, a 15-minute standard regenerative BISA vibration training is performed. There is no regenerative vibration training done after the second test.

Conclusion: The optimal effect of the regenerative BISA vibration training on the reduction of cortisol levels within 45 minutes is clearly recognizable. The second test without BISA vibration training showed no reduction in cortisol levels even after 45 minutes of intensive exertion from running.

A reduced cortisol level subsequently is the ideal prerequisite for rapid replenishment of the glycogen stores in the liver and muscles. However, this extraordinary effect with the aid of SALUSSTAR® Innoplate vibration technology works only if the athletes have a sufficient micronutrient supply.

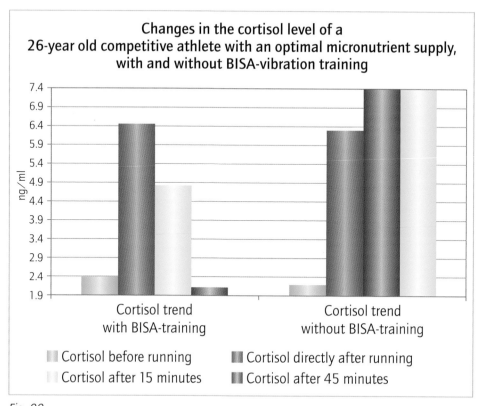

Fig. 99

Appendix

Table 29: Micronutrient dosage recommendations for recreational and competitive athletes in terms of customized micronutrient formulations, based on results from our intracellular blood tests, nutrition analyses, protocol sheets and other criteria (see pg. 171, fig. 72) compared to previous DGE (German Nutrition Society) guidelines, which are also the

Vitamins	Important metabolic function in sports	Recommended supply/day (DGE: Adult)[3]	Food sources
Vitamin C Ascorbic acid, water-soluble	• Carnitine-biosynthesis • Stress-resistance neurotransmitter balance • Antioxidative cell protection • Iron utilization • Protection of vessels (endothelium) • Hormone metabolism	100 mg	• Kiwi • Broccoli • Peppers
Vitamin B₁ Thiamine, water-soluble	• Mental capacity • Energetic utilization of carbohydrates (mitochondria) • Heart, nerve, and muscle metabolism	1.2 mg for athletes 0.5 mg/1,000 kcal energy turnover	• Grain germ • Soy flour • Pork • Bran • Vegetables • Nuts • Organ meats
Vitamin B₂ Riboflavin, water-soluble	• Antioxidative cell protection • Stabilization of the immune system	1.4 mg for athletes 0.6 mg/1,000 kcal energy turnover	• Wheat germ • Wheat bran • Dairy products • Grains

guidelines of the German Society for Sports Medicine and Prevention (DGSP). An interpretation of the micronutrient analyses is not based on individual element concentrations but rather on deviation from the respective median value of results from 9,150 top and 6,434 recreational athletes.

Possible symptoms of an under-supply	Optimal micronutrient concentration through blood tests serum/plasma[1, 6] excretion/urin[6] intracellular[1] (in erythrocytes)	Dosage recommendations: performance-oriented recreational athlete[2] (endurance athletes with up to 6 h training)	Dosage recommendations: performance and top athletes[2]
• Limited stress resistance and regeneration • Susceptibility to infection • Muscle weakness • Pain in limbs and joints • Lack of motivation, concentration and poor performance Irritability	Plasma/serum: good supply: [2, 6] Recreational athletes: > 70-85 µmol/l Performance athletes: > 90-170 µmol/l Top athletes: 150-200 µmol/l	500-1,500 mg	500-3,000 mg (also intravenously in cases of infections and sports injuries)
• Limited stress resistance and regeneration • Susceptibility to infection • Muscle weakness • Pain in limbs and joints • Insomnia • Irritability • Loss of appetite • Lack of motivation, concentration and poor performance	Intracellular (in ery.)[1] Deficient <73 µg/l ery. Optimal: 20% above median value	5-30 mg[4]	10-70 mg[4]
• Susceptibility to infection • Lack of motivation, concentration and poor performance • Muscle weakness	Intracellular (in ery.)[1] Deficient < 380.1 µg/l ery. Optimal: 20% above median value	10-40 mg[4]	20-70 mg[4]

Vitamins	Important metabolic function in sports	Recommended supply/day (DGE: Adult)[3]	Food sources
Vitamin B3 niacin/ niacinamide, water-soluble	• Antioxidative cell protection • Stabilization of the immune system • Mitochondrial energy metabolism	13-17 mg niacin equivalent = 60 g tryptophan for athletes 6.6 mg/1,000 kcal energy turnove	• Meat, fish • Organ meats • Dairy products • Grains
Vitamin B5 pantothenic acid, water-soluble	• Carbohydrate, fat and protein utilization • Synthesis of stress hormones • Availability of acetyl-CoA (universal metabolic building block)	6-10 mg	• Fish • Mushrooms • Legumes
Vitamin B6 pyridoxine	• Immune competence • Regulation of amino acid metabolism (protein formation) • Neurotransmitter synthesis • Glycogen metabolism • Homocysteine detoxification	1.4-1.5 mg for athletes: depending on protein intake: = 0.15 mg/mg protein/day	• Whole grain products • Yeast • Fish • Poultry
Vitamin B9 folic acid, water-soluble	• Energy metabolism • Protein formation • Cell regeneration (mucous membranes) • DNA formation • Nerve formation and protection	0.4 mg folate equivalent	• Leafy green vegetables • Whole grains

Possible symptoms of an under-supply	Optimal micronutrient concentration through blood tests serum/plasma[1, 6] excretion/urin[6] intracellular[1] (in erythrocytes)	Dosage recommendations: performance-oriented recreational athlete[2] (endurance athletes with up to 6 h training)	Dosage recommendations: performance and top athletes[2]
• Susceptibility to infection • Loss of appetite • Muscle weakness • Lack of motivation, concentration, and poor performance	Vitamin B$_3$-status:[6] relationship of renal excretion of N-methyl-2-pyridone-3-carboxamide and n-methylnicotinamide in urine normal: 1.3-4.0; deficiency < 1.0	10-30 mg	20-60 mg[4] athletes with skin allergies may have a reaction with doses of > 30 mg
• Limited stress resistance and regeneration	Pantothenic acid status in urine[6] normal level > 1mg/d	10-40 mg	20-80 mg[4]
• Susceptibility to infection • Limited stress resistance and regeneration • Muscle weakness • Insomnia • Loss of appetite • Irritability • Lack of motivation, concentration, and poor performance	Intracellular (in ery.) Deficient: < 215 µg/l ery. Optimal: 20% above median value	5-30 mg	10-80 mg[4]
• Limited stress resistance and regeneration • Susceptibility to infection • Muscle weakness • Insomnia • Irritability • Lack of motivation, concentration, and poor performance	Intracellular (in ery.) Deficient: < 796 µg/l ery. Optimal: > 20% above median value	0.4-1.2 g	0.8-1.6 g[4]

Vitamins	Important metabolic function in sports	Recommended supply/day (DGE: Adult)[3]	Food sources
Vitamin B$_{12}$ cobalamine	• Energy metabolism • Nerve formation and protection • Blood formation (hematopoiesis) • Cell regeneration • DNA formation	3.0 µg	• Liver • Dairy products • Fish • Eggs
Vitamin H biotin, water-soluble		30-60 µg (assessed value for adequate supply)	• Organ meats • Peas • Nuts
Vitamin D[5] califerol, fat-soluble	• Bone metabolism • Calcium absorption and utilization • Muscle contraction • Strengthening of the immune system	5-10 µg (200-400 i. u.)	• Ocean fish • Veal • Mushrooms • Egg yolk • Butter • Hard cheese • To convert vitamin D-precursor: sunlight

Possible symptoms of an under-supply	Optimal micronutrient concentration through blood tests serum/plasma[1, 6] excretion/urin[6] intracellular[1] (in erythrocytes)	Dosage recommendations: performance-oriented recreational athlete[2] (endurance athletes with up to 6 h training)	Dosage recommendations: performance and top athletes[2]
• Susceptibility to infection • Lack of motivation, concentration, and poor performance • Irritability • Muscle weakness • Limited stress resistance and regeneration • Insomnia	Serum concentration:[1] intracellular not measurable because fluctuation is too great. Deficient: < 700 µg/ ml Optimal: 20% above median value	20-60 µg	30-400 µg[4]
• Muscle aches • Limited stress tolerance and regeneration • Lack of motivation, concentration, and poor performance	Biotin excretion in urine:[6] 25-50 µg/24 h	45-100 µg	45-200 µg
• Susceptibility to fatigue fractures • Muscle weakness • Susceptibility to infection • Delayed regeneration • Poor bone density and osseous weight bearing capacity	Vitamin D-status:[1, 6] 25-OH vitamin D_3 in serum: Deficient: < 80 nmol/l Optimal: 20% above median value	400-1,000 i. u. per day, particularly in fall and winter, for indoor sports a good calcium supply is especially important.	400-1,000 i. u. per day, particularly during fall and winter, a good calcium supply is especially important for all indoor sports

Vitamins	Important metabolic function in sports	Recommended supply/day (DGE: Adult)[3]	Food sources
Vitamin A[5] retinol, fat-soluble	• Formation and preservation of mucous membranes • Strengthening of immune defense • Antioxidative protection • Hormone metabolism	0.8-1 mg (2,500-3,500 i. u.)	• Cod liver oil • Organ meats • Eggs • Dairy products
Vitamin E (alpha, gamma tocopherol, etc.)	• Antioxidative protection • Regulation of immune system and inflammation metabolism • Protection of vessels	12-15 mg tocopherol equivalent, or 18-22 i. u. (assessed value for an adequate supply)	• Olive oil • Wheat germ oil • Walnuts
Vitamin K phylloquinone	• Bone metabolism • Bone formation • Blood formation and clotting	60-80 µg (assessed value for an adequate supply)	• Leafy green vegetables • Sauerkraut

[1] Customized micronutrient formulations are based on results from intracellular blood tests, additional measured parameters, results from nutrition analysis and a protocol sheet.

[2] Dosages that have verifiably reduced the athletes' injury and infection risk.

[3] The previously recommended supply is only derived from basic considerations on the relationship between energy use and increased nutrient requirements. The listed recommendations are joint recommendations from German-speaking nutrition societies (Germany, Austria, Switzerland). To date there is a vast lack of sports-medical performance-physiological data for the practical review of the clinical relevance of previous dosage recommendations.

Possible symptoms of an under-supply	Optimal micronutrient concentration through blood tests serum/plasma[1, 6] excretion/urin[6] intracellular[1] (in erythrocytes)	Dosage recommendations: performance-oriented recreational athlete[2] (endurance athletes with up to 6 h training)	Dosage recommendations: performance and top athletes[2]
• Susceptibility to infection • Limited capacity • Delayed regeneration	Serum level (good supply):[6] >30 µg/dl Interpretation of serum values is difficult due to retinol homeostasis.	0.8-1 mg 2,500-3,500 i. u.	1-3 mg 2,500-10,000 i. u. Performance should not take more than 10,000 i. u. long-term; sensible for endurance athletes with frequent upper respiratory infections.
• Poor performance • Muscle aches • At risk for oxidative muscle damage • Impaired regeneration ability • Susceptibility to infection	Vitamin E-(alpha-tocopherol) status:[2, 6] Plasma concentration Deficient < 3.8 µmol/l Optimal: 20% above the median value	150-250 mg 275 i. u.-375 i. u.	200-400 mg 300 i. u.-600 i. u.
	Vitamin K status[6] Plasma: normal value um 1.0 nmol/l	60-150 µg	150-500 µg (caution when taking blood-thinning medications)

[4] Athletes with skin problems (such as acne, neurodermatitis, psoriasis) in some cases may experience a worsening of the complexion with an increase of some B-vitamins.
Notes: Targeted intravenous therapies in cases of exhaustion are not taken into consideration here, but they can be implemented by attending physicians in individual cases after a specific diagnosis.

[5] Vitamin A and D should not exceed the listed reference values.

[6] Specifications by Gröber from *Metabolic Tuning statt Doping* – Hirzel Publishing 2008 and *Mikronährstoffe* – Scientific Publishing Company Stuttgart, 2nd edition 2006.

Table 30: Micronutrients dosage recommendations for recreational and competitive athletes in terms of a customized micronutrient formulation, based on the results from our intracellular and other blood tests, nutrition analyses, an additional protocol sheet and other criteria (see pg. 171, fig. 72) as compared to the previous DGE (German Nutrition

Vitaminoids	Important metabolic function in sports[3]	Recommended supply/day (DGE: Adult)[3]	Food sources
L-carnitine	• Energy production from fats (mitochondria and fatty acid transport)	Approx. 100 mg (DGE: no recommendation)	• Lamb • Beef
Coenzyme Q_{10}	• Antioxidants, stabilization of cell membranes • Cellular energy production	Unknown	• Olive oil • Eggs • Liver
Alpha-lipoic acid	• Energy production from carbo-hydrates (in conjunction with B_1)	Unknown	–
Omega-3 fatty acids	• Building block for each cell membrane • Immune stabilization • Anti-inflammatory • Increases mental capacity and ability to concentrate • Improved oxygen supply to organs	Unknown	• Oil from ocean fish (herring, wild salmon) • Soy oil • Corn oil • Fish oil usually contains approx. 30-35% Omega-3 fatty acids

[1] Customized micronutrient formulations are based on results from intracellular blood tests, additional measured parameters, results from nutrition analysis and a protocol sheet.

[2] Dosages that have verifiably reduced the athletes' injury and infection risk.

[3] The previously recommended supply is only derived from basic considerations on the relationship between energy use and increased nutrient requirements. The listed recommendations are joint

Society) guidelines, which are also the guidelines of the German Society for Sports Medicine and Prevention (DGSP). An interpretation of the micronutrient analyses is not based on individual element concentrations but rather on deviation from the respective median value of results from 9,150 top and 6,434 recreational athletes.

Possible symptoms of an under-supply	Optimal micronutrient concentrations via blood tests serum/plasma[4, 1] whole blood, intracellular	Dosage recommendations: performance-oriented recreational athlete[2] (endurance athletes with up to 6 h training)	Dosage recommendations: performance and top athletes[2]
• Impaired fat and carbohydrate metabolism • Susceptibility to infection • Fatigue	Free carnitine (FC) in plasma: 40-60 µmol/l Ratio of acylcarnitine/ f0ree carnitine AC/FC-quotient: normal or good supply: Fasting: < 0.7 Postprandial: < 0.4	250-1,000 mg	1,000-3,000 mg
Not yet known	In whole blood: Deficient: < 1.5 mg/l cholesterol-corrected < 0.2 µmol/mmol Optimal: 20% above median value	30 mg	30-150 mg
Not yet known		60-200 mg	200-400 mg
• Limited stress tolerance • Poor mental capacity and ability to concentrate • Increased danger of damage to cell membranes • Increased susceptibility to infection	Optimal diagnostics membrane lipids in the ery. Serum: alpha-linoic acid: Deficient: < 30 mg/l Deficient EPA: < 30 mg/l DHA: < 110 mg/l Optimal: 20% above median value	0.5-1 g Information: 1 g (omega-3 fatty acid = approx. 3 g fish oil) (High concentrates contain 85%)	1-3 g Information: 1g (omega-3 fatty acid = approx. 3 g fish oil) (High concentrates contain 85%)

recommendations from German-speaking nutrition societies (Germany, Austria, Switzerland). To date there is a vast lack of sports medical performance physiological data for the practical review of the clinical relevance of previous dosage recommendations.

[4] Specifications by Gröber from *Metabolic Tuning statt Doping* – Hirzel Publishing 2008 and *Mikronährstoffe* – Scientific Publishing Company Stuttgart, 2nd edition 2006.

Table 31: Micronutrients dosage recommendations for recreational and competitive athletes in terms of a customized micronutrient formulation, based on the results from our intracellular and other blood tests, nutrition analyses, an additional protocol sheet and other criteria (see pg. 171, fig. 72) as compared to the previous DGE (German Nutrition

Minerals	Important metabolic function in sports	Recommended supply/day (DGE: Adult)[3]	Food sources
Calcium	• Stabilization of cell membranes • Important tasks in heart, nerve and muscle function • Stabilization of bone structure	1,000-1,200 mg	• Dairy products • Green cabbage
Magnesium	• Carbohydrate, fat and protein metabolism • Activation of more than 300 enzymes (important to energy metabolism • Stabilization of cell membranes • Calcium antagonist	300-400 mg	• Specific mineral waters • Whole grain • Bananas • Nuts
Potassium	• Short-term replenishment of carbohydrate stores in liver and muscles • Acid-base balance • Stimulation of nerves and muscles • Impulse conduction in cardiac muscle	2,000 mg (assessed value for minimum supply)	• Bananas • Potatoes • Vegetables • 100% fresh pressed juices • Wheat germ

Society) guidelines, which are also the guidelines of the German Society for Sports Medicine and Prevention (DGSP). An interpretation of the micronutrient analyses is not based on individual element concentrations but rather on deviation from the respective median value of results from 9,150 top and 6,434 recreational athletes.

Possible symptoms of an under-supply	Optimal micronutrient concentrations via blood tests serum/plasma[4] intracellular[1]	Dosage recommendations: performance-oriented recreational athlete[2] (endurance athletes with up to 6 h training)	Dosage recommendations: performance and top athletes[2]
• Increased neuroexcitability • Muscle twitches • Cramps (tetany)	Calcium status:[4] serum concentration 2.2-2.65 mmol/l (= 8.8-10.6 mg/dl	200-400 mg	400-700 mg
• Increased susceptibility to stress • Overexcitability • Poor regeneration • Cramps • Lid and muscle twitches • No optimal development of endurance capacity	Intracellular (in ery.):[1] Deficient: < 50 mg/ery. Optimal: 20% above median value	200-400 mg Optimal for athletes as orotate chewable tablets 35 mg Another possibility: aspartate, citrate	300-600 mg Optimal for athletes as orotate chewable tablets 35 mg Another possibility: aspartate, citrate
• Muscle weakness • Loss of appetite • Poor regeneration • Cardiac arrhythmia	Optimal intracellular:[1] Technically hardly feasible, since the blood can only be transported in a frozen state. Alternative: Whole blood for athletes Deficient: < 1.798 mg/l Optimal: 20% above median value	100-300 mg 150-300 mg/l during exertion phase as an electrolyte beverage	500-1,000 mg Especially in endurance sports during regeneration phase

Minerals	Important metabolic function in sports	Recommended supply/day (DGE: Adult)[3]	Food sources
Sodium, chloride	• Regulation of water and electrolyte balance • Preservation of membrane potential	2,000 mg sodium 3,000 mg chloride	• Cooking salt • Mineral water
Iron	• Oxygen supply to organs, blood formation • Enzyme component (for energy supply)	10-15 mg	• Meat • Chanterelle mushrooms • Unsulphured apricots • Blueberry extract

Trace elements	Important metabolic function in sports	Recommended supply/day (DGE: Adult)[3]	Food sources
Iodine	• Energy balance • Formation of thyroid hormones	150-200 µg	• Ocean fish • Iodized salt

Possible symptoms of an under-supply	Optimal micronutrient concentrations via blood tests serum/plasma[4] intracellular[1]	Dosage recommendations: performance-oriented recreational athlete[2] (endurance athletes with up to 6 h training)	Dosage recommendations: performance and top athletes[2]
• Increased tendency to cramps • Insufficient regeneration after athletic exertion • Dizziness	Serum/plasma:[4] 136-145 mmol/l	2,000-3,000 mg sodium 3,000-4,000 mg chloride	3,000-6,000 mg sodium 4,500-9,000 mg chloride
• Fatigue • Poor regeneration • Prevents optimal performance development • Dizziness • Pale complexion • Nervousness • Hair loss	Serum ferritin:[1] optimal for endurance athletes Men > 70 µg/l Women > 50 µg/l	10-100 mg[1] taken only after blood test and with doctor's orders	10-100 mg[1] taken only after blood test and with doctor's orders

Possible symptoms of an under-supply	Optimal micronutrient concentrations via blood tests serum/plasma[4] intracellular[1]	Dosage recommendations: performance-oriented recreational athlete[2] (endurance athletes with up to 6 h training)	Dosage recommendations: performance and top athletes[2]
• Poor performance • Night sweats • Increased fatigue • Lack of motivation • Lack of concentration ability • Poor regeneration after exertion • Struma formation	Iodine status: excretion in urine between 100-150 µg/d > 100 µg/g creatine	100-200 µg (if there is no exercise-induced increase in TSH > 2.5 µIU/l, a specific iodine supply should be given initially.)	100-300 µg (if there is no exercise-induced increase in TSH > 2.5 µIU/l, a specific iodine supply should be given initially.)

Trace elements	Important metabolic function in sports	Recommended supply/day (DGE: Adult)[3]	Food sources
Zinc	• Immune stabilization • Supports numerous functions in carbohydrate, fat and protein metabolism • Insulin storage	7-10 mg	• Oysters • Cheese • Legumes • Beef fillet
Selenium	• Regulation of thyroid hormones • Antioxidants • Immune stabilization	30-70 µg (assessed value for an adequate supply)	• Whole grain (products) • Ocean fish • Liver
Chromium	• Fat metabolism • Optimizes replenishment of glycogen stores	30-100 µg	• Meat • Cheese • Mushrooms • Brewers yeast

Possible symptoms of an under-supply	Optimal micronutrient concentrations via blood tests serum/plasma[4] intracellular[1]	Dosage recommendations: performance-oriented recreational athlete[2] (endurance athletes with up to 6 h training)	Dosage recommendations: performance and top athletes[2]
• Allergic reactions • Increased incidents of pollen allergies • Increased susceptibility to infection • Hair loss • Inhibited sense of taste and smell	Intracellular (in ery.)[1] Deficient: < 14 mg/l ery. In athletes with pollen allergy < 15 mg/ ery. Optimal: > 20% above median value	10-30 mg Short-term in cases of current infections	20-50 mg Short-term in cases of current infections
• Increased susceptibility to infection • Inhibited thyroid function	Intracellular (in ery.)[1] Deficient: < 114.4 µg/l ery. Optimal: > 20% above median value	50-150 µg	100-200 µg Long-term use of more than 200 µg can have toxic effect.
• Inhibited glucose utilization in energy production and fat metabolism	Whole blood status:[2, 4] < 90 µmol/l Serum: 13 mmol/l Reference values show significant differences. Optimal: 20% above median value	50-150 µg	100-300 µg

Trace elements	Important metabolic function in sports[3]	Recommended supply/day (DGE: Adult)[3]	Food sources
Copper	• Iron transport • Immune stability • Blood formation • Collagen and neurotransmitter synthesis	1-1,5 mg	• Nuts
Manganese	• Carbohydrate metabolism • Antioxidants • Bone and cartilage growth	2-5 mg	–

Possible symptoms of an under-supply	Optimal micronutrient concentrations via blood tests serum/plasma[4] intracellular[1]	Dosage recommendations: performance-oriented recreational athlete[2] (endurance athletes with up to 6 h training)	Dosage recommendations: performance and top athletes[2]
• Increased rate of infection • Anemia • Fat metabolism • Brittle bones	Copper status: serum:[4] Men: 80-130 µg/dl Women: 75-120 µg/dl (urine: 10 µg/24 h) During acute or chronic infections the serum copper level is often elevated. Whole blood status:[2] Deficient: < 0.7 mg/l Optimal: > 20% above median value	2-4 mg	4-8 mg An optimal zinc/copper ratio is an important prerequisite for appropriate absorption from the gastrointestinal tract.
• Inhibited carbohydrate metabolism • Suppression of bone and cartilage growth	Reference range: Deficient: Whole blood: < 7.0 µg/l Optimal: 20% above median value	5-10 mg	10-20 mg

[1] Customized micronutrient formulations are based on results from intracellular blood tests, additional the measured parameters, results from nutrition analysis and a protocol sheet.

[2] Dosages that have verifiably reduced the athletes' injury and infection risk.

[3] The previously recommended supply is only derived from basic considerations on the relationship between energy use and increased nutrient requirements. The listed recommendations are joint recommendations from German-speaking nutrition societies (Germany, Austria, Switzerland). To date there is a vast lack of sports medical performance physiological data for the practical review of the clinical relevance of previous dosage recommendations.

[4] Specifications by Gröber from *Metabolic Tuning statt Doping* – Hirzel Publishing 2008 and *Mikronährstoffe* – Scientific Publishing Company Stuttgart, 2nd edition 2006.

Table 32: Micronutrients dosage recommendations for recreational and competitive athletes in terms of a customized micronutrient formulation, based on the results from our intracellular and other blood tests, nutrition analyses, an additional protocol sheet and other criteria (see pg. 171, fig. 72) (dosages are equivalent to 30-70 g of an AM-formula

Amino acids	Important metabolic function in sports	Recommended supply/day (DGE: Adult)[3]	Food sources
Arginine, conditionally essential	• Energy metabolism • Regeneration after exertion important to formation of connective tissue • Immune systemstimulation • Release of growth hormone	–	• Fish • Meat • Soy products • Whole rice • Peanuts • Almonds
Glutamine	• Immune stability • Energy production • Stabilization of blood sugar level • Regeneration	–	• Whole grain products • Soy products • Daily products
Glycine, conditionally essential	• Immune system stimulation • Formation of immunoglobulin • Detoxification of the liver	–	• Beef • Gelatin

blend, see pg. 173, table 9). A suggested dose of this AM-formula blend is not based on the individual element concentrations, but rather on deviation from the respective median value (adequate supply equals > 20% of the assessed median value) of results from 9,150 top and 6,434 recreational athletes.

Possible symptoms of an under-supply	Optimal micronutrient concentrations via blood tests serum/plasma[4]	Dosage recommendations: performance-oriented recreational athlete[2] (endurance athletes with up to 6 h training)	Dosage recommendations: performance and top athletes[2]
• Weakened immunity (increased infections) • Increased risk of injury to many connective tissue structures (tendon-ligament apparatus, etc.)	Serum/plasma: Deficient: < 2.2 mg/dl Optimal: > 20% above median value	3 g	3-7 g
• Decrease in physical capacity • Increased susceptibility to infection • Inhibited intestinal function	Serum/plasma: Deficient: < 9.8 mg/dl Optimal: > 20% above median value	2-4 g	4-10 g
• Inhibited immune system • Increased risk of injury to many connective tissue structures (tendons, ligaments, etc.)	Serum/plasma: Deficient: < 2.8 mg/dl Optimal: > 20% above median value	6-10 g	6-14 g

Amino acids	Important metabolic function in sports	Recommended supply/day (DGE: Adult)[3]	Food sources
Leucine/ isoleucine Valine, essential branched-chain amino acids	• Energy production • Protection from premature fatigue Regeneration	Leucine: 14 mg/kg body weight Isoleucine: 10 mg/kg of body weight Valine: 14 mg/kg of body weight	• Legumes • Oats • Potatoes • Whole grain products • Parmesan cheese • Eggs • Meat • Rice • Dairy products
Lysine, essential	• Immune system stimulation • Collagen synthesis • Carnitine synthesis • Formation of connective tissue structures	10 mg/kg of body weight	• Potatoes • Wheat • Soy products • Eggs (egg whites) • Meat
Methionine, essential, sulphurous amino acid	• Formation of many connective tissue structures (tendons, ligaments etc.) • Formation of glutathione (together with cysteine) • Formation of coenzyme Q_{10} for synthesis of CP-stores	13 mg/kg of body weight	• Lentils • Soy products • Low-fat dairy products • Eggs • Fish

Possible symptoms of an under-supply	Optimal micronutrient concentrations via blood tests serum/plasma[4]	Dosage recommendations: performance-oriented recreational athlete[2] (endurance athletes with up to 6 h training)	Dosage recommendations: performance and top athletes[2]
• Rapid physical and mental fatigue • Muscle weakness • Inhibited ammonia detoxification	Serum/plasma: Deficient: Leusine: < 3.3 mg/dl Isoleucine: < 2.2 mg/dl Valine: < 4,1 mg/dl Optimal: > 20% above median value	Leucine: 2 g Isoleucine: 1.5 g Valine: 2 g	Leucine: 2-4 g Isoleucine. 1. 5-3 g Valine: 2-4.4 g
• Increased susceptibility to infection • Increased susceptibility to injury of many connective tissue structures (tendons, ligaments etc.) • Inhibited carnitine and fat metabolism	Serum/plasma: Deficient: < 3.4 mg/dl Optimal: > 20% above median value	1 g	Up to 2.5 g
• Decreased immune function • Increased susceptibility to injury of many connective tissue structures • Poor regeneration after sprints	Serum/plasma Deficient: < 0.9 mg/dl Optimal: > 20% above median value	0.2 g	Up to 0.4 g

Amino acids	Important metabolic function in sports	Recommended supply/day (DGE: Adult)[3]	Food sources
Taurine, conditionally essential	• Stabilization of the immune system • Strong antioxidant	–	• Organ meats • Meat extracts • Meat
Tryptophan, essential	• Formation of hormones serotonin, melantonin, and vitamin niacin	3 mg/kg body weight	• Bananas • Soy • Lentils • Peanuts • Parmesan cheese • Dairy products
Cysteine, glutathione, conditionally essential, sulphurous amino acids	• Immune competence • Protection of cells from free radicals • Glutathione synthesis (together with methionine)	–	• Corn • Oats • Eggs (egg whites) • Green vegetables (spinach, broccoli etc.) • Asparagus

Possible symptoms of an under-supply	Optimal micronutrient concentrations via blood tests serum/plasma[4]	Dosage recommendations: performance-oriented recreational athlete[2] (endurance athletes with up to 6 h training)	Dosage recommendations: performance and top athletes[2]
• Inhibited immune function • Oxidative stress	Serum/plasma: Deficient: > 3.2 mg/dl Optimal: > 20% above median value	0.2-0.4 g To date we have not given additional taurine.	0.4-0.8 g To date we have not given additional taurine.
• Sleep disturbance • Bad mood • Depressed mood	Serum/plasma: Deficient: < 2.0 mg/dl Optimal: > 20% above median value	500 mg separate supply in the evening, two hours before bedtime.	500-1,000 mg separate supply in the evening, two hours before bedtime.
• Inhibited immune function • Oxidative stress • Formation of many connective tissue structures (tendons, ligaments etc.)	Plasma/serum: Deficient: < 1.8 mg/dl Optimal: > 20% above median value	0.5-1 g cysteine as n-acetyl cysteine[4] separately, as needed	1-2 g cysteine as n-acetyl cysteine[4] separately, as needed.

[1] Customized micronutrient formulations are based on results from intracellular blood tests, additional measured parameters, results from nutrition analysis and a protocol sheet.

[2] Dosages that have verifiably reduced the athletes' injury and infection risk.

[3] The previously recommended supply is only derived from basic considerations on the relationship between energy use and increased nutrient requirements. The listed recommendations are joint recommendations from German-speaking nutrition societies (Germany, Austria, Switzerland). To date there is a vast lack of sports medical performance physiological data for the practical review of the clinical relevance of previous dosage recommendations

[4] Specifications by Gröber from *Metabolic Tuning statt Doping* – Hirzel Publishing 2008 and *Mikronährstoffe* – Scientific Publishing Company Stuttgart, 2nd edition 2006.

Table 33: The common nutrition importance of amino acids

Amino acids (essential, semi-essential)	Special characteristics	Especially plentiful in:
Leucine (essential)	• Boosts protein synthesis (protein anabolism) • Inhibits breakdown of muscle protein (catabolism). • Emergency energy carrier for muscle cells. • Counteracts excessive serotonin formation (less fatigue in situations of particular exertion). Caution: As a nutritional supplement leucine should only be taken together with isoleucine and valine, otherwise the protein synthesis may be impaired.	• Whey protein • Oat protein • Corn protein • Millet protein • Egg protein • Casein • Free in cocoa • Hazelnut protein
Isoleucine (essential)	• Boosts protein synthesis. • Emergency energy carrier for muscle cells. • Counteracts excessive serotonin formation (s. a.).	• Lactalbumin • Casein • Meat protein • Egg protein • Hazelnut protein
Valine (essential)	• Emergency energy carrier for muscle cells. • Counteracts excessive serotonin formation (s. a.).	• Lactalbumin • Casein • Oat protein • Meat protein • Egg protein • Hazelnut protein • Whole rice protein
Phenylalanine (essential)	• Precursor substance for the activating neurotransmitter dopamine. • A specific supply may decrease formation of the fatigue-causing neurotransmitter serotonin. • Since dopamine is formed by the intermediate stage tyrosine, the assessment of a protein should be based on the sum of both amino acids.	• Applies to phenylalanine and tyrosine: casein • Hazelnut protein • Whole rice protein • Peanut protein • Albumen protein
Tryptophan (essential)	• Precursors of the calming neurotransmitter serotonin; specific supply promotes sleep-readiness. • Important for vitamin synthesis in the body (niacin). • Tryptophan is destroyed during technical hydrolysis of protein and is thus absent in gelatin hydrolysates.	• Lactalbumin (as part of whey protein) • Cashew protein • Whey protein • Albumen protein
Threonine (essential)	• Easily used for energy production during major physical exertion. • Particularly high threonine requirements during anabolic phases.	• Whey protein • Egg yolk protein • Pea protein • Wheat germ protein • Beef protein

Amino acids (essential, semi-essential)	Special characteristics	Especially plentiful in:
Histidine (semi-essential)	• Important for the formation of blood pigment hemoglobin. • Is more easily excreted in urine than any other amino acid. Since zinc that is bound to histidine is lost in this process, taking high doses of histidine should be avoided. • As a supplement it should boost blood clotting. • Contrary to other amino acids, only about 60% is absorbed in the intestinal tract. • Can boost protection of cells.	• Banana protein (8%) • Tuna protein • Mackerel protein • Beef protein
Lysine (essential)	• Mostquality-limiting amino acid in vegetarian foods. • Becomes indigestible when heated to high temperatures, which is why baked goods usually contain very little lysine. • Starting substance for the body's natural carnitine. • Lysine content and thereby wheat protein valence diminish with intensive fertilization. • The extremely low lysine content in cornflakes gives them practically no a nutritional standpoint.	• Lactalbumin • Casein • Egg protein • Meat protein • Soy protein • Potato protein • Amaranth protein • Wheat protein • Lentil protein • Free in potato water
Methionine (essential)	• Intensifies the effects of arginine. • Supplies sulphur for many syntheses of the body's natural substances. • Supplies methyl groups for syntheses. • Particularly high requirements during anabolic phases. • Improves wound healing. • Facilitates formation of cysteine and taurine in the body. • The sum of methionine and cysteine is pivotal to the assessment of proteins. • Breakdown of methionine produces "sulphuric acid"; more base foods (vegetables, fruit, magnesium citrate) should be consumed to avoid hyperacidity from a diet that is high in methionine.	• Applies to: the sum of methionine and cysteine: • Albumen protein • Whole egg protein • Fish protein • Liver protein • Oat protein • Brazil nut protein • Whole corn protein

Amino acids (essential, semi-essential)	Special characteristics	Especially plentiful in:
Arginine (essential)	• Important to liver metabolism (urea formation, ammonia breakdown) • Particularly important during the early regeneration phase after intensive physical exertion. • Improves anabolic utilization of milk protein (low in arginine) at least 4 g for 100 g Casein, 5 g for 100 g whey protein, 1.5 g arginine for 1l of milk. • In the body arginine is quickly converted to ornithine and vice-versa. Therefore arginine can be largely substituted by ornithine. From a nutrition-physiological-standpoint the sum of arginine and ornithine is pivotal. • Improves protein synthesis (anabolism) in higher quantities and also with increased release of growth hormones. As little as 3 g can be effective when taken on an emptystomach. • Local use is particularly effective in boosting decreasing hair growth. • Boosts immune system, e.g. in an over-trained athlete – may cause activation of "dormant" herpes viruses and may be irritating. • Improves fat metabolism and can lower blood cholesterol concentration. • Larger amounts can have a diuretic effect (if so, supply should be split into smaller portions). • Precursor for nitrogen oxide (NO) that functions as an antioxidant and boosts circulation by widening peripheral vessels.	• Almonds 14.8 g • Walnuts 14.6 g • Peanuts 13.8 g • Coconut 12.6 g • Meat/fish and soy protein 7-8 g/100 g • Whole rice protein 8.3 g/100 g • Oat protein 7.3 g/100g
Ornithine (semi-essential)	• Basically like arginine since it is quickly converted to arginine in the liver as well as reconverted to ornithine (urea cycle). • When taking higher quantities it is wise to take a mix of arginine and ornithine (2:1). • For physiological reasons it is also expedient to simultaneously take lysine, e.g. arg./orn./lys. ratio of 2:1:0.5. • Persons with renal insufficiency should avoid a supply of Arg/Orn.	• Liver

Amino acids (essential, semi-essential)	Special characteristics	Especially plentiful in:
Tyrosine (semi-essential)	• Precursor to activity-boosting neurotransmitter dopamine. • Specific supply can have stimulating effect. • From a nutrition-physiological standpoint the sum of phenylalanine and tyrosine is pivotal since tyrosine forms from phenylalanine. • Individuals with kidney disease may produce so little natural tyrosine that a nutritional supplement with tyrosine is important. • Tyrosine has poor water-solubility and is therefore hardly useable in liquid preparations.	• Casein • Whole milk protein • Pea protein • Egg yolk protein • Peanut protein • Bean protein
Cysteine (semi-essential)	• Important to the secondary structure of many proteins due to the formation of sulphur bridges. • A genetically high cysteine level is the reason for curly or frizzy hair. • Nutritional supplements containing cysteine will boost hair growth. • From a nutrition-physiological standpoint the sum of methionine and cysteine is pivotal since 2/3 of the required methionine supply can be taken in the form of cysteine (also see methionine). • Cysteine occurs in the blood primarily as a double cysteine molecule. • Cysteine has poor water-solubility and is therefore hardly useable in liquid preparations. • Cysteine is necessary for glutathione syntheses, which is important for protection of cells against free radicals (e.g. during athletic activity).	• Albumen protein • Oat protein • Whole corn protein
Proline (semi-essential)	• Proline particularly important for formation of connective tissue protein: hydroxyproline released through the breakdown of connective tissue cannot be reused for buildup and must be excreted in urine. • During an energy shortage large amounts of proline are used for energy production, such as during long fasts or athletic endurance performances. • Free Proline is in considerable quantity in fruit juice (example up to 2,5 g per l orange juice).	• Casein • Whole milk protein • Wheat germ protein

Amino acids (essential, semi-essential)	Special characteristics	Especially plentiful in:
Alanine (non-essential)	• In catabolic situations transports amino groups from muscle to liver (urea synthesis) • Helps form glucose in the liver (gluconeogenesis) during glucose shortages or stress metabolism. • During intensive physical exertion significant amounts of alanine are used after the first hour. • Alanine replacement is wise after exertions of more than one hour. • Alanine can also boost the protein synthesis in the liver.	• Gelatin (9.8%) • Whole corn protein • Beef protein • Albumin protein • Pork protein • Rice protein • Soy protein • Oat protein
Glycine (semi-essential)	• As the most basic of all amino acids it is the universal supplier of amino groups for the synthesis of other substances, e.g. blood pigment hemoglobin. • Important to the connective tissue protein synthesis. • High glycine requirements during anabolic phases. • Danger of connective tissue protein breakdown with insufficient supply. • High glycine supply inhibits the protein-catabolizing enzyme cathepsin D and decreases the breakdown of connective tissue in catabolic situations (preserves the barrier function of connective tissue against penetrating germs). • Glycine has cell-protecting properties during temporary oxygen shortages.	• Gelatin (23.8%) • Beef protein • Liver protein • Peanut protein • Oat protein
Serine (non-essential except in cases of kidney failure)	• Normally can be easily formed from glycine (mainly in the kidneys) with the use of methionine, e.g. from methionine and vice-versa. • From a nutrition-physiology standpoint the sum of both amino acids is pivotal because of the close link between serine and glycine.	• Egg yolk protein • Albumen protein • Casein • Whey protein • Oat protein • Corn protein
Aspartic acid (non-essential)	• Vital function in energy metabolism as well as the liver. • Supports ammonia detoxification via the urea cycle in the liver. • Very important is a supply early in phase of regeneration normalizing the ammoniak concentration. • Produced in the body among other things through the decomposition of Aspargin.	• As aspartic acid and asparagine: • Potato protein (20.7%) • Coconut protein (17.1%)

Amino acids (essential, semi-essential)	Special characteristics	Especially plentiful in:
	• Free in many fruit juices and vegetables (together with asparagine): passion fruit 1.6 g/ l • Food ingredient charts list aspartic acid plus asparagine	• Alfaalfa protein (12.3%) • Peanut protein • Albumen protein • Meat protein
Asparagine (non-essential)	• Close metabolic relationship with aspartic acid. • Contrary to aspartic acid appears to be of little significance in the human organism. • Occurs in many fruit, berry and vegetable juices as free amino acid; apple juice can contain approx. 1g/l.	
Glutamic acid (non-essential)	• Important transfer point for amino nitrate in metabolism. • Forms during breakdown of some amino acids as intermediate stage, particularly proline, histidine, arginine and ornithine. • In spite of regeneration a large amount of the free glutamic acid supply is lost during intensive endurance workouts. For this reason a supply of these amino acids is important after endurance workouts. • Can bind ammonia with the formation of glutamine and transport it to the liver, which turns it into urea and glucose; boosts arginine's ammonia-reducing effect. • Boosts protein formation – likely the reason for high glutamic acid content in milk. • In the form of sodium salt ("glutamate") most commonly used seasoning in the world. • The previously assumed increase in brain capacity is very controversial. • As far back as 1953, Dr. Nöcker described a beneficial effect on physical capacity. • Excessive individual doses can cause nausea (Chinese restaurant syndrome) in particularly sensitive individuals, probably due to a vitamin B_6 deficiency. • For reasons of technical analysis only the sum of glutamic acid and glutamine is known for most foods. • In several food there is available the arid form of Pyroglutamin acid (potato).	• White flour protein • Whole wheat protein • Caspein • Potato protein • Hazelnut protein • Pork protein • Whole rye protein • Whey protein • Beef protein • Soy protein

Amino acids (essential, semi-essential)	Special characteristics	Especially plentiful in:
Glutamine (essential in stress metabolism)	• In terms of quantity the most important amino acid in the body. • Forms from glutamic acid through reaction with ammonia. • Most important energy carrier for some cells, such as mucosa cells (in small intestine) and cells of the immune system. • Stimulates glycogen synthesis (as a wheat flour component it is important for the benefits of "pasta loading" before a competition). • Improves protein synthesis in catabolic metabolism situations. • Regulates muscle protein synthesis (probably by stabilizing water balance in the cell). • Essential in catabolic metabolism situations. • A few important foods also contain a lot of glutamine (more than glutamic acid). The 20-24% glutamic acid content of milk protein listed on food labels in reality is based 2/3 on glutamine since it only turned into glutamic acid during the analysis stage. • Some foods also contain significant amounts of free glutamine: tomatoes (0.65%), potato water and other vegetables. • Large amounts of glutamine can be lost during intensive athletic exertion. Quick replenishment benefits regeneration and assures the anabolic training effect. • Glutamine is necessary for the formation of glutathione, which is important for the protection of cells from free radicals (e.g. athletic activity).	• Wheat protein (up to 30%) • Oat protein • Casein • Whey protein
Taurine (amino acid-like and essential in infants and in catabolic metabolism situations – also in sports)	• Stable end product of sulphurous amino acid metabolism. • Important for the stabilization of the cells' water balance and thus for protein synthesis. • Vital for the development of an infant's brain. • Has properties that protect the cell membrane, and is thus useful during intensive athletic exertion. • Acts as catcher of radicals and protects the cell from damage during particular stress.	• Meat extract • Meat • Mussels

Amino acids (essential, semi-essential)	Special characteristics	Especially plentiful in:
	• Has regulating function in heart muscle and therefore is considered as stress protection for the heart in Japan (is consumed in large quantities there as a heart protection soft drink). • Boosts formation and effectiveness of bile (taurocholic acid) as emulsifier in fat digestion. • Prevents over-stimulation of nerves from caffeine – thus increases the safety of caffeinated beverage consumption (also in sports). • Has no stimulating effect. • Can increase transportability of fat-soluble foreign substances in the body and boosts their excretion.	

Photo: Jupiterimages

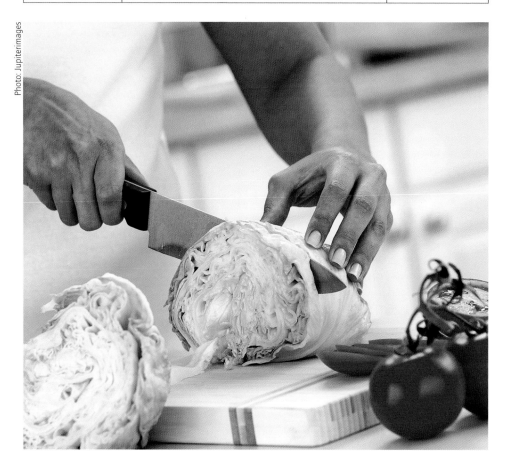

Master copy drink log

Name:				
Date	Time	Quantity	Beverage	Place
	6:00 am			
	7:00 am			
	8:00 am			
	9:00 am			
	10:00 am			
	11:00 am			
	12:00 pm			
	1:00 pm			
	2:00 pm			
	3:00 pm			
	4:00 pm			
	5:00 pm			
	6:00 pm			
	7:00 pm			
	8:00 pm			
	9:00 pm			
	10:00 pm			
	11:00 pm			
	12:00 am			
	Daily total	Liters		
	Still need	Liters		

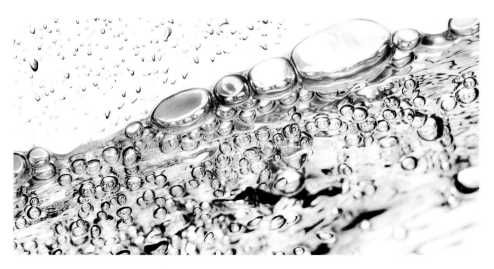

For information and dissemination

Competitive athletes, trainers, physical therapists, etc., can download all of the following charts as PDF-files from the publisher's website with the user name "explosion and the following code number: xutRZ4qt

Subject fluid balance

Effective drinking with base beverages

Mineral water: sodium content > 350 mg, but less than 1,000 mg

The higher the bicarbonate concentration of mineral water (hydrogen carbonate), the more easily excess acid is transferred into the blood.

Bicarbonate concentration: minimum > 500 mg
Optimal > 1,500 mg of still water without carbonation

Drinking sodium-rich fluids in sports

- Rapid carbohydrate absorption

- Rapid water absorption

- Minimal urinary excretion

Fig. 100

Faster recovery with smart eating and drinking after sports

Fast regeneration happens through targeted replenishment
of glycogen stores in the liver and muscles
during the first two hours after exertion.

**Phase 1 directly after competition or training.
Regeneration beverage: recovery drink**

• do not drink more than 500 ml at a time – otherwise it is badly absorbed.

• Carbohydrate content 35-70 g per l (approx. 3-7%)
all drinks over 6% stop the speed of gastric emptying
e.g. Cola with 11%

• Sodium content over 350 mg/per l
(1 effervescent Kalinor tablet from the pharmacy 750 mg)

• Supplement or mix with a good still mineral water.

• Protein content of approx. 20-25 g per l
(supplement with 2 Tbs AM-formula blend dissolved in 250 ml of juice)

Fig. 101

Important drinking tips

• Once you're thirsty, it's too late.

• Gradually increase fluid amounts so the gastrointestinal tract
can adjust to the increased amounts of fluid.

• The gastrointestinal tract cannot absorb fluid
amounts of > 500 ml.

• Pay attention to the quality of mineral waters as described.

• Taking magnesium during athletic exertion is not sensible
because it puts too much strain on the gastrointestinal tract,
which can lead to intolerance.

Fig. 102

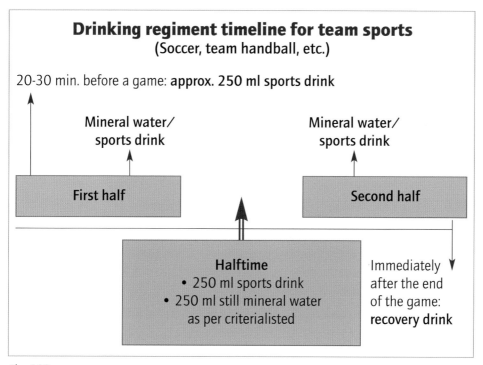

Drinking regiment timeline for team sports
(Soccer, team handball, etc.)

20-30 min. before a game: **approx. 250 ml sports drink**

| Mineral water/ sports drink | | Mineral water/ sports drink |

| **First half** | | **Second half** |

Halftime
- 250 ml sports drink
- 250 ml still mineral water as per criterialisted

Immediately after the end of the game: **recovery drink**

Fig. 103

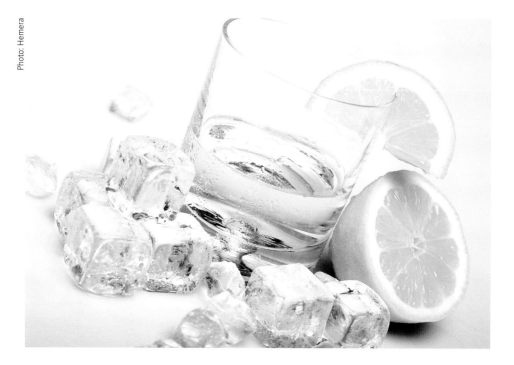

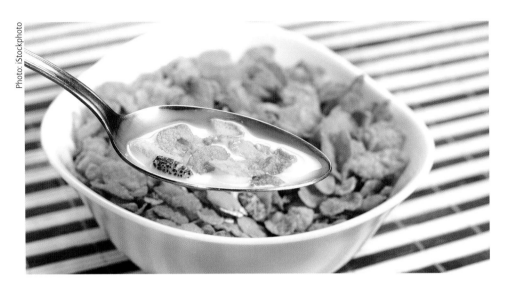

Photo: iStockphoto

Subject nutrition

The primary goal should not be gambling away victory, but rather achieving improved performance through specific nutrition tips and better recovery. We offer practical recommendations for breakfast, lunch and dinner combinations.

Meals on a training day

Get-fit breakfast
(High in carbohydrates)

• 5 Tbs Quaker oats (whole oats, whole grain cereal)

• 3 Tbs Wheat germ, 1 banana, sliced,
yoghurt (also vanilla yoghurt)
and 1 glass of fresh pressed orange juice.

First training:
During training drink approx. 500 ml (sports drink mixed
with a high-quality mineral water as described)
(Optimal sodium-hydrogen carbonate content).

Immediately after training:
2-3 heaping Tsp AM-formula blend,
e.g. dissolve in 200 ml juice, stir and drink
(Replenishes amino acid pools and stabilizes connective tissue).

Fig. 104

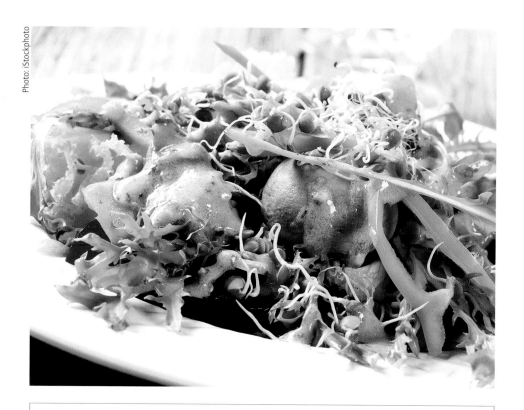

Photo: iStockphoto

Lunch
From the accompanying carbo-loading chart
(Beneficial food combinations)

Optimal and fast recovery with carbohydrates, potassium, chromium
and a high-quality protein combination

Example:
- 3-4 potatoes
- 125 g curd cheese with herbs, seasonal herbs, salt and pepper
- Salad of seasonal greens with fresh champignon mushrooms
- 1-2 eggs
- Dessert: 1/2 fresh pineapple
or a small fruit salad (kiwi, bananas, etc.)

Afternoon
High-quality granola bars, fruit tart, etc., for inbetween.

Fig. 105

Evening
Carbo-loading from the skillet (pasta or rice and vegetables)
Easy meal to prepare at home

Optimal and fast recovery with carbohydrates, potassium, chromium
and a high-quality protein combination.
Whole grain pasta or wild rice contains silica –
stabilization of tendons and ligaments.

- 150 g wild rice or whole grain pasta, cook for 15 min.
- Put approx. 150 g of frozen vegetables in a skillet
with 1 Tbs oil
and the wild rice or pasta.
Cook and stir 6-8 min.
- Dessert: Curd cheese with fruit.

Fig. 106

Helpful hints

- 1-2 hours prior to exertion: e.g white bread with lots of honey
or jam, without butter.
- Add mild, ripe, base-friendly fruit:
well suited are melon, mango or pear
– no unripe fruit – because it stays in the stomach too long.
- No competition/training without breakfast –
better to get up early
- Practice more effective drinking – only then will you be able
to implement this in a competition.
- Eating oranges, kiwi, grapefruit every day
keeps your connective tissue young.
- Pack fruit every day as a snack.
- Avoid lots of sweets, white flour products (white pasta, white rice),
a lot of meat and cold cuts, as these make your metabolism too
acidic and block absorption of important micronutrients.
- The first two hours after exertion
determine your regeneration time
(optimal behavior-particularly in terms
of diet-ensures success.)

Abb. 107

Literary references

Billigmann, P. & Siebrecht, S. (2004). *Physiologie des L-Carnitins und seine Bedeutung für Sportler.* Hannover: Schlüterische Verlagsgesellschaft.

Bruyere, O. et al. (2004). Glucosamine sulfate reduces osteoarthritis progression in postmenopauspausal women with knee osteoarthritis: evidence form two 3-year-studies. *Menopause*, 11, 138-143.

Ders. et al. (2002). Evaluation des Magnesiumstatus bei Ausdauersportlern. *Deutsche Zeitschrift für Sportmedizin*, 3, 72.

Ders. (2006). *Mikronährstoffe in der orthomolekularen Medizin.* Stuttgart: Wissenschaftliche Verlagsgesellschaft.

DGE (Deutsche Gesellschaft für Ernährung, Hrsg.). (2004). *Ernährungsbericht 2004.* Frankfurt am Main.

DGE (Deutsche Gesellschaft für Ernährung, Hrsg.). (2005). *Kleine Nährwerttabelle,* 43. überarbeitete und aktualisierte Auflage.

Dickhuth, H.-H., Mayer, F., Röcker, K. & Berg, A. (Hrsg.). (2007). *Sportmedizin für Ärzte.* Köln: Deutscher Ärzte-Verlag.

Faude, O., Fuhmann, M., Herrmann, M., Kindermann, W. & Urhausen, A. (2005). *Ernährungsanalysen und Vitaminstatus bei deutschen Spitzenathleten. Leistungssport* (19.5.2005).

Fenech, M. & Ferguson, L. R. (2001). *Mutations-Research.* 475, 1-283.

Feil, W. & Wessinghage, Th. (2005). *Ernährung und Training.* Nürnberg: WesspVerlag.

Friedrich, W (2006). *Optimale Sporternährung.* Spitta Verlag.

Geiss, K.-R. et al. (1994). Steigerung der Ausdauerleistungsfähigkeit durch Magnesiumorotat bei Ausdauersportlern. *Der Kassenarzt,* 20, 40-41.

Geyer, H. et al. (2004). Analysis of non-hormonal nutritional supplements for anabolic-androgenic steroids – results of an international study. *Int J Sports Med,* 25(2), 124-129.

Gröber, U. (2008). *Metabolic Tuning statt Doping – Mikronährstoffe im Sport.* Stuttgart: Hirzel-Verlag.

Gröber, U. (2006[2]). *Mikronährstoffe.* Wissenschaftliche Verlagsgesellschaft Stuttgart.

Ho, J. Y. et al. (2010). *Metabolism.* in Press.

Kraemer, J. W. et al. (2005). *Chem Month, 136* (8),1383.

Mao, I. F. et al. (2001). Elektrolyt loss in sweat and iodine deficiency in a hot environment. *Arch Enviorn Health*, 56 (3), 271-277.

Matheson, A. J., Perry, C. M. (2003). Glucosamine: review of it use in the management of osteoarthritis. *Drugs Aging, 20*, 1041-1060.

Maughan, R. J., Burke, L. M. & Cooyle, E. F. (Eds.) (2004). *Food, nutrition and sports Performance II.* The international Olympic Committee Consensus on Sports Nutrition. London.

Müller, D. M. et al. (2002). *Metabolism, 51* (11), 1389.

Neidhart, M. et al. (2000). Increased serum levels so non-collagenous matrix proteins (cartilage oligometric matrix protein and melanoma inhibitory activity) in marathon runners. *Osteoarthr. & Cart, 8,* 222-229.

Saur, P. (2004). Magnesium und Sport. *Deutsche Zeitschrift für Sportmedizin, 55* (1), 23-24.

Schek, A. (2/2005). *Top-Leistung im Sport durch bedürfnisgerechte Ernährung.* Münster/Westf.: Philippka Sportverlag.

Spiering, B. A. et al. (2007). *J Strength Cond Res, 21* (1), 259.

Dies. (2008). *J Strength Cond Res, 22* (4),1130.

Volek, J. S. et al. (2002). *Am J Physiol Endocrinol Metab, 282*, E474.

Wienecke, E. (2005). *Fit für freie Radikale. Einfach gesund.* Weil der Stadt: Hädecke.

Ders. (2007). Advances in Therapy – *The International Journal of Drug, Device and Diagnostik Research.* (September/Oktober).

Wutzke, K. D. et al. (2004). *Metabolism, 53* (8), 1002.

Acknowledgements

Words of gratitude

Successful visionary concepts are only possible with good partners. Many thanks to Prof. Dr. med. Reiner Körfer and his team, particularly Dr. Heinrich Körtke, who have played a pivotal role in SALUTO's advancement.

Special thanks goes to the Bertelsmann Foundation, especially to Liz Mohn, whose past screening campaign provided a crucial foundation for today's successful Anti-Doping Concept with its revolutionary findings in the area of micronutrient therapy in competitive athletes.

A sincere thank you to Gerhard Weber, Udo Hardiek and Ralf Weber who contributed to SALUTO's progress with their life's work, GERRY WEBER World (stadium, sports park, hotel, event center), and supported us through the years. We look forward to our continued successful collaboration.

About SALUTO

SALUTO (Society for Sport and Health)

SALUTO was launched at the University Bielefeld, Germany in the area of sports science, especially the department of sports medicine. Prof. Dr. Elmar Wienecke is the founder and owner. A combination of medical services, diagnostics, science and research has helped SALUTO evolve into an internationally recognized center of excellence for health and fitness within the world of GERRY WEBER in Germany.

Over a period of 15 years, SALUTO, in cooperation with the HDZ (Heart and Diabetes Center) and the IDPE (dental practices) developed integrated survey designs that helped competitive and elite athletes from all sports achieve international success.

Clinical studies and numerous research projects on individual micronutrient requirements have resulted in the establishment of a one-of-a-kind European database of 6,434 leisure and 9,150 elite athletes, that is based on a specially designed technique for cellular analyses (www.saluto.de).

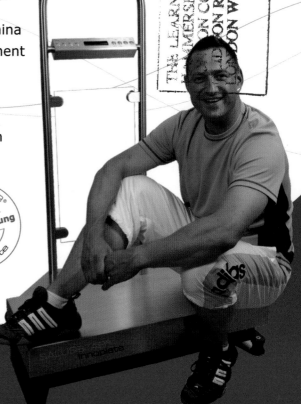

Appendix

Customized micronutrient formulations by SALUTO are composed according to the criteria listed on page 171, fig. 72.

Important building blocks are:

The "Unique Building Block System" by HCK®	Amino acids	L-carnitine

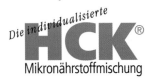

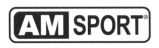

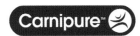

Carnipure™ bietet reinstes L-Carnitin und ist ein Warenzeichen der Lonza AG, Schweiz.

www.hepart.com
www.unisan.de

www.amsport.de

www.carnipure-for-you.com

Other partners:

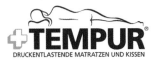

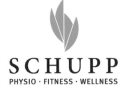

SALUTO
DAS KOMPETENZZENTRUM FÜR GESUNDHEIT UND FITNESS IN DEUTSCHLAND

www.tempur.de

www.schupp-gmbh.de

www.saluto.de

Photo Credits:

Cover design: Sabine Groten

Cover photo: dpa, Picture-Alliance/photographer Faugere Franck

Photos (inside): see individual photos

Illustrations: Pg. 37, 42, 54, 57,60, 123 Corinna Reinders (Meyer & Meyer Publishing); Background **images:** mycola/Thinkstock, Jupiter Images/Thinkstock

Pg. 61: Illustration: National Institutes of Health, US Dept. of Health and Human Services, taken from http://en-wikipedia.org/wiki/file:skeletal_muscle.png
Pg. 63: Illustration: from Gray's Anatomy:
http://upload.wikimedia.org/wikipedia/commons/b/b8/Lumbricales_pedis.png
Pg. 66: Illustration: Mysid/UweGille: from
http://upload.wikimedia.org/wikipedia/commons/b/be/Knee_diagram-de.svg
Pg. 67: Illustration: Rene Gräber, taken from:
http://upload.wikimedia.org/wikipedia/de/2/2c/Kniegelenkvorne.jpg
Pg. 69: Illustration; debivort, taken from:
http://commons.wikimedia.org/wiki/File:ACDF_oblique_blank.png
Pg. 81: Illustration: Tatoute, taken from: http://commons.wikimedia.org/wiki/File:Mitochondrie.svg

All other illustrations: www.satzstudio-hilger.de